pulse

voices from the heart of medicine

The first year

Voices from the Heart of Medicine, Inc.
28 Albert Place
New Rochelle, NY 10801
USA

www.pulsemagazine.org

ISBN - 13: 978 0 6155533 5 1

Typset by Pindar NZ, Auckland, New Zealand

Cover and interior graphic design by
Laurie Douglas Graphic Design (www.lauriedouglas.com)

Original edition published by cChange in Healthcare Publishing

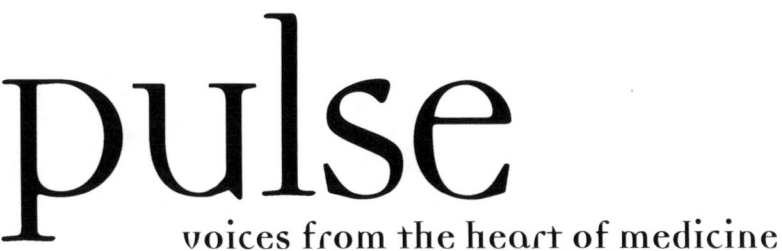

pulse
voices from the heart of medicine

The first year

Paul Gross MD and Diane Guernsey
With a Foreword by Peter Selwyn MD MPH

Poetry Editors:
Judy Schaefer RNC MA and Johanna Shapiro PhD

Senior Poetry Consultant: Jack Coulehan MD MPH

Story Editors: Diane Guernsey, Beth Hadas, Warren Holleman PhD, Barry Jacobs PsyD, David Loxterkamp MD, Jo Marie Reilly MD, Amy Selwyn, Joanne Wilkinson MD MSc, and Neal Whitman EdD

contents

acknowledgments

Pulse—voices from the heart of medicine, this book and the web site (www.pulsemagazine.org), would never have come into being without the help and guidance of many individuals—and some institutions.

Sy Safransky's magazine *The Sun* was an inspiration: It showed us that a publication of personal experiences could not only exist, it could be extraordinary.

Long before *Pulse* had a name, Larry Bauer of the Family Medicine Education Consortium was the first to listen and offer much-needed encouragement.

In spring 2005 a group of people that included Larry, Peter Selwyn, Julie Schirmer, Andrea Gordon, Joanne Wilkinson, Jo Marie Reilly, Colleen Fogarty, Stuart Green, Lu Marchand and Craig Irvine met in New Orleans at the annual meeting of the Society of Teachers of Family Medicine to bat around the idea of a magazine of personal health care experience. This gathering evolved into the *Pulse* Advisory Group. They became a sounding board for everything from Pulse's name, suggested by Warren Holleman, to its content, shaped by Sayantani DasGupta, who persuaded us that *Pulse* would become a more unique and forceful publication if it welcomed every voice in health care to its pages.

Over time, the *Pulse* Advisory Group grew further to include the following friends: Ashrei Bayewitz, Cortney Davis, Mary Duggan, Ronit Fallek, Laravic Flores, Lana Guernsey, Jonathan Han, David Loxterkamp, Maggie Mahar and Dan O'Connell.

Each of them has contributed far more to *Pulse* than he or she realizes.

We owe a debt to Kevin Shanley, a knowledgeable and committed magazine consultant who, in carefully outlining for us the steps—and finances—of launching a print publication, helped us to see that our path forward lay on the Web.

We thank Micah Sifry, who drew on his own writing and publishing experiences to make the case that the Web was *Pulse*'s natural medium.

Special thanks go to Pamela Fiori, editor-in-chief of *Town & Country* magazine, and Janet Carlson, *Town & Country*'s health and beauty director, for their generous attentiveness and encouragement, and for spreading the word about *Pulse* in the pages of *Town & Country*.

To our parents, siblings, in-laws and children, who have followed *Pulse*'s progress with interest (and a tinge of bemusement), we offer our deep thanks for your tolerance and support.

We're deeply grateful to two institutions—Albert Einstein College of Medicine and Montefiore Medical Center—for welcoming new ideas, caring about compassionate health care and valuing the humanistic education of their medical students and residents. Among *Pulse*'s many friends and allies in the Department of Family and Social Medicine and the Residency Program in Social Medicine, Administrator Mona Weinberger stands out for her unfailing kindness and support, as does Program Development Director Paul Meissner for keeping us focused on *Pulse*'s financial needs and potential.

At Einstein, we would particularly like to single out Al Kuperman, associate dean of medical education, who championed *Pulse* in its earliest days and who for years has been an inspiration and ally to teachers and advocates of medical humanism. We'd also like to acknowledge Karen Gardner, Einstein's manager of internal and Web communications, who was quick to appreciate *Pulse*'s possibilities and eager to promote it within and outside the institution.

At Montefiore, it is no small gift that hospital President Steven Safyer is an avid *Pulse* reader and supporter. And Anne McDarby, Montefiore's manager of public relations, has become an invaluable friend.

In any endeavor there are those upon whose shoulders the entire enterprise rests. At *Pulse*, these shoulders belong to:

Pulse's writers, who have turned their personal experiences into compelling stories and moving poems, who have entrusted their creative efforts and egos to us, and who have responded appreciatively to our editorial suggestions.

Pulse's unfailingly kind and sensitive editors, who have so generously lent us their time and talents and have worked collaboratively with our writers to set a high literary standard for *Pulse*'s offerings.

The renowned physician-poet Jack Coulehan, who asked, sight unseen, what he could do to help bring *Pulse* to life.

Johanna Shapiro and Judy Schaefer, two gifted poets and editors who agreed, without ever having met us and before a single issue of *Pulse* had seen the light of day, to sign on as *Pulse*'s poetry editors—a rash act for which we will always be grateful. For their poetic and editorial talents, for their leadership and generosity, and for their unfailing sensitivity, kindness and good humor, we thank them.

Laurie Douglas, a uniquely gifted and experienced graphic designer, who was recommended by a colleague at a time when we thought that *Pulse* would materialize on paper. After designing a logo and a number of covers for a never-to-be-realized print version, Laurie shifted gears without a hitch and created *Pulse*'s Web site's graphics. She also designed the book you are now holding. Laurie's visuals have brought energy, pizzazz and credibility to our project, and for this we are inexpressibly grateful.

Stephen Yorke, the highly experienced Web developer we enlisted once we decided that *Pulse* would be a Web-based publication. To Stephen fell the task of designing and erecting a user-friendly site that would welcome a growing list of subscribers while simultaneously making it easy for a couple of rookies to produce and distribute a weekly issue of *Pulse*. Luckily, he was more than up to the task. For his patient willingness to explore every nuance of the project, for his expertise, for his commitment to meeting our needs, and for succeeding brilliantly—we thank him.

And finally, Peter Selwyn, chair of the Department of Family and Social Medicine at Montefiore and Albert Einstein, who, when first discussing Paul's coming to work for him, listened respectfully to the vaguely formulated notions that would evolve into *Pulse* and, rather than nodding politely and moving on to something more realistic, suggested that he might be able to provide support for such an undertaking. Peter's understanding, encouragement, kindness, humor and practical backing—and the personal example he sets as an enormously gifted physician-writer—have inspired us and made *Pulse* a practical reality. Our gratitude is deeper than words can express.

Paul Gross MD and Diane Guernsey

for our daughters, cara and aster, with all our love

foreword

It has become popular in medical education to refer to the emerging field of "narrative medicine," which it is hoped will help humanize the process of becoming a doctor and increase physicians' self-awareness beyond their standard professional roles. Though such a hope may seem farfetched, I believe that narrative medicine—essentially, telling and listening to stories—does have this power.

In a sense, narrative medicine's pull lies in its ability to connect us to much earlier times in human history, well before the emergence of medicine itself. For millennia, people have come together, in countless venues and circumstances—around campfires, dinner tables, tribal talking circles and other gathering places—to share the stories of their lives. Telling your story to others, listening to theirs, remembering, bearing witness and appreciating each other's experiences are among the deepest fundamentals of human communication.

In medicine, both patient and caregiver come to the medical encounter with their own history, experiences and "baggage"—their stories. Sharing these can help us to recognize our common humanity and, in profound ways, open the door to healing for patient and caregiver alike. How does this happen?

Empathy, another term now popular in medical education, cannot be formally taught, yet it is indispensible to the daily work of any physician who interacts with patients. Empathy begins when we can keep our hearts open to other people's experiences, emotions and perceptions so that we feel some of what they feel, by connecting these to our own experience or history.

As physicians, we enjoy the great privilege of witnessing people's lives in intimate and unguarded detail every day, and we also bear the great responsibility of taking this witness and using it to form healing relationships in which we can offer our patients the help they most deeply need. Listening empathically to our patients' stories, and letting our own stories percolate up through us into consciousness, enables us to do this.

Empathy also teaches us as much about ourselves as it does about the people with whom we interact. At the end of the day—as at the end of life and other human milestones—the distinctions between doctor and patient fall away, and we realize that we are all traveling the same human path. This realization—that we're not alone—is itself profoundly healing.

Several years ago, I was very pleased to help Paul Gross take the first steps toward establishing *Pulse*. Since then, I've found it rewarding to watch this interesting and speculative idea evolve into a compelling reality, involving not only Paul but also a committed and talented Editorial Board, a growing circle of dedicated writers and a readership that has expanded to more than 4,000 people since its launch in 2008. *Pulse* has provided a virtual gathering place where the members of our collective modern tribe—all of us who are affected in some way by the healthcare system—have been able to come together to share our stories.

This first year's collection is breathtaking in the range of circumstances and characters it depicts and in its depth of emotion, courage and honesty of self-reflection, and concise clarity of expression. I find it gratifying that many of *Pulse*'s contributors are clinicians in practice, and inspiring to read the stories of those contributors who have been patients or caregivers. At the same time, I know that these distinctions are often arbitrary—we are all in this together. *Pulse* shines a light on our common humanity as we all make our way along the trail. Thanks again to *Pulse*'s writers for being our guides. I am proud to be part of this expedition.

Peter A. Selwyn MD MPH
Professor and Chairman
Department of Family and Social Medicine
Montefiore Medical Center
Albert Einstein College of Medicine
Bronx, NY

introduction

Pulse—voices from the heart of medicine is the work of many people. It has probably meant something different to each of them. For me, *Pulse* grew out of a search for truth.

A similar search for truth—applied to the human body—brought me into medicine in the first place. How does the body work? What causes it to malfunction? How can we fix it when it's broken?

After more than a decade of practice as a family doctor, I came to appreciate that the science I'd learned in medical school, though powerful and useful, was also incomplete. Like many comprehensive systems aimed at explaining our world, it contained much truth about illness and healing, but not the whole truth.

Clinical studies told me that my patient Mrs. Ortiz might benefit from daily doses of calcium to strengthen her bones. But these studies couldn't tell me whether it made sense to actually prescribe it when Mrs. Ortiz was already shaking her head at the eleven pills she had to swallow each day for her high blood pressure, diabetes and cholesterol.

And although in medical school I'd learned the names of neurotransmitters that might be involved in depression, my learning didn't cover the pain that another patient, Mrs. Reyes, had felt when she'd emigrated to the United States from the Dominican Republic, leaving her young daughter behind. Nor did it address whether an antidepressant pill—assuming she could tolerate it—would actually help someone in her situation.

My patients, I found, had thoughts, feelings, personalities, life experiences and family members that deeply influenced their symptoms and their interest in my prescriptions.

Not only that, my patients had a doctor who had thoughts, feelings and life experiences of his own. He had his good days and his bad days. He had two delightful daughters and a talented, caring wife who also wanted and needed his love and attention. He felt upset and thrown off balance when things didn't go well—whether at home or in the office.

His patient encounters were filled with small dramas that, as he tried to apply the textbook medicine he'd learned, not infrequently ended in farce. His life as a physician bore little resemblance to the doctor shows on television. There were no chest compressions here, no urgent dashes to the OR. And his patients never played starring roles in the case studies he read about in medical journals.

I concluded that these medical journals might help me become a better doctor in the same way that studying a psychology textbook might help a shy teenager get ready to ask a secret crush out on a date.

Yes, these articles contained truths that, when artfully applied, could cure illness and save lives. But they were silent on the practical issue of how to apply these truths in the real world of crowded waiting rooms and fifteen-minute visits—a matter as critical as knowing what to say after your crush answers the phone.

For me, it was precisely here that the practice of medicine came alive. Depending on the day, I could take part in situations that were perplexing, humorous or heartbreaking—or all three. And if these complex situations never made their way into medical journals, they did provide great material for stories—the kind that I shared with colleagues, with my wife and with friends—sometimes accompanied by laughter, a rueful shake of the head or even a welling of the eyes.

I discovered that writing and sharing my healthcare stories with others was therapeutic. Doing so allowed me to turn my hurts and triumphs into something potentially beautiful, funny or moving.

I also came to realize that there were others in health care who felt as I did—and that I got just as much out of reading their stories as I did from sharing my own.

Why did I find these stories so compelling?

They affirmed my own experience; they told me that I wasn't alone.

They portrayed health providers as the real people we are—vulnerable and conflicted at times, but also principled and courageous. In their honesty and warmth they offered a lesson to all of us, including the students whom we hope to train to be humane professionals.

These stories provided a forum for patients who wanted to tell us about their journeys through illness—and to teach us how to give them better care.

They showed patients that healthcare providers are mortals whose power to cure is often limited, but whose wish to heal runs deep.

And they revealed a healthcare system that is complex and disorganized—and sometimes cruel and unfair.

As I was mulling over the power of stories and poems to hurt or heal, the talk of healthcare reform was gathering momentum. It seemed like the right time to share these stories so that we all—patients, caregivers and health professionals—could let our aspirations guide us in our search for a better way to deliver health care.

And so, in early 2008, with the help of a group of dedicated and supportive colleagues across the country, *Pulse—voices from the heart of medicine* was launched, a modest publication consisting of a Web site (www.pulsemagazine.org) and software that enabled us to e-mail one story or poem each week to a national—and international—readership.

My Advisory Board colleagues and I made some crucial editorial decisions early on:

Pulse stories had to be first-person. They needed to be true, and they needed to recount the writer's own experience.

We decided that *Pulse* should invite the participation of every person involved in health care—including patients, doctors, nurses, caregivers, mental-health professionals and staff.

Since part of *Pulse*'s mission was to foster understanding, we decided that *Pulse*'s stories and poems needed to use clear, simple language. No medical jargon. No arcane literary devices. If *Pulse* was to encourage dialogue, we had to make sure that any reader could understand it.

And while *Pulse* had a lofty mission—to foster a dialogue that could change health care—we also knew that it would only succeed if it entertained and engaged its readers and left them wanting more.

Not a medical journal . . . not a literary magazine. What was it? A newsletter? Too dull. An e-zine? Too techno.

In the end, we decided to call *Pulse* an online magazine—one that arrived on your virtual doorstep, like a real magazine. But, unlike a print magazine, each issue would consist of only one story or poem, making *Pulse* rather like a banquet comprised of bite-sized courses.

The first issue of *Pulse* was sent out to 2,100 subscribers on April 13, 2008, a Sunday. Our weekly publication day soon shifted to Friday, an upbeat time for readers winding down from a hectic work week. For many, we learned, *Pulse*'s arrival became a welcome signal of the weekend's approach.

This volume contains all of the stories and poems that appeared in *Pulse*'s first year—from April 13, 2008 to April 17, 2009. They are arranged in chronological order and grouped by season, beginning with family doctor Joanne Wilkinson's powerfully self-revealing "Well Baby Check" and finishing with ER nurse Stacy Nigliazzo's moving encounters with the extremes of life in "Coming Full Circle."

I hope that this will be the first of many yearly *Pulse* anthologies. I hope, too, that readers will be touched and entertained, that some will use this book to teach their students about two values that we in medicine hold dear—humanism and professionalism—and that others will share it with friends and relatives to let them know what it's really like being a health professional, a health-professional-in-training or a patient.

I hope that people will pass this book around because everyone loves a good story or poem—particularly when the drama of illness is involved.

Finally, I hope that some readers will feel inspired to jot down and share their own experiences in health care and their encounters with our current health system, whose power to shape our medical experiences has yet to be fully appreciated. It is our belief that these yet-to-be-written stories may prove to be critical in leading health care into a new, more enlightened age.

Paul Gross MD
New Rochelle, NY

spring

well baby check

Joanne Wilkinson
4/13/2008

I get to clinic early today, undaunted by the double- and triple-bookings in my schedule. "We have a baby coming today," I tell the medical assistant. "A new baby. Six pounds. Born yesterday. Bring him right back when he comes."

I miss seeing newborns in the office; I had a lot of babies in my practice as a resident. Now I see a patient population that is half hardscrabble Spanish-speaking diabetics with back pain, and half blonde twenty-three-year-old medical students on the pill. I haven't seen a newborn in two years. But last year, one of the medical students had the kind of textbook pregnancy that twenty-four-year-olds can have sometimes. It was a marked contrast from the medicated, bed-resting, amniocentesis-punctuated pregnancies my forty-year-old friends have endured this year, and I am eager to see her, and her baby boy.

This fall my husband and I decided to adopt. We had discovered, through "pre-conception" blood work, the presence of a factor that could increase my risk for blood clots. That alone might not have deterred me, but there were other, scarier factors: My mother's early death from a heart attack when I was nine. The fact that I have hypertension, just as she did. The likelihood that her heart attack was caused by a similar blood clot, and the fact that I am exactly the same age that she was when she died. In the end, we decided not to tempt fate, and bought a book about China instead.

The torrent of unwanted advice we received from our peers was astounding. Co-workers and acquaintances who barely knew my husband's name nevertheless felt free to offer their opinions. I would "regret" not having "my own," I was told. I simply couldn't imagine, they said, how wonderful it felt to have "your own." I would always wonder what if, they told me, then made the ominous Adoption Pronouncement: "You just don't know what you're getting that way." I would watch these people's mouths move as they spoke, recalling my tenth year, when teachers and grown-ups would tell me that surely my mother couldn't be dead. "Oh, you mean your grandmother," more than one said when I tried to explain. I would blink silently back, amazed at the conviction of a person who could tell a ten-year-old that she was mistaken about whether her parents were alive.

I stopped trying to explain myself to these people, but I knew they inhabited a different reality than mine. In their world, the sun shone brightly and little girls sometimes got confused about why their mother hadn't contributed to the bake sale. I know the people trying to tell me when and how I should become a mother are in a parallel universe, wondering why my planet can't get with the program and join their orbit. I can't explain to them that I link becoming a mother with dying, that I would rather never have children than have a child like me, left alone as a little girl. I know what I know, but still they are able to make me feel bad, and when they open their mouths to give the advice, I feel myself shrink inside.

I can't find the strength to deal with these people, but I can tell others to do it: Megan, the medical student, and her husband e-mailed me last month about circumcising their baby. They had thought about it and decided they were interested, but the midwife at their birthing center had spent fifteen minutes telling them how unnatural it was, and now they were unsure. I told them what I always tell my new parents. "This is your kid. You get to decide. You're the mommy and daddy now. Don't let anyone give you any shit." As I press send, I realize that I am going to be a mommy someday, and I need to start listening to my own advice.

Here come the mommy and daddy now. Their six-pound day-old infant looks like a compact burrito with a head of wild dark hair. He's calm, and sucks my pinky finger furiously when I listen to his lungs. His little legs bicycle aimlessly in the air as I examine his tummy. I have been gradually preparing myself for what my childbirth will be like—not the drumbeat of the fetal monitor, not the pushing, the crying, the new life slick with blood and fluid, but instead the paperwork, the plane flight, the strange country smelling of spices we don't use, and the weight in my arms of a six-month-old, a nine-month-old, a bigger kid who doesn't look like me. I think of my child, my future abstract baby, and already feel sad that I will not have the chance to hold her during her first day in the world. I cup my hands behind this baby's fragile skull, glad for the chance, at least, to hold this one. Then I hand Megan's little bundle back to her and tell her what she already knows, that he is perfect.

About the author: Joanne Wilkinson MD MSc decided to be a doctor when she was eight so that she could support her writing habit. "I told my pediatrician that I was going to be a writer, but that in order to make money I would be a doctor 'during the day.' He laughed ... now I know why." Since then, Joanne has attended and led multiple writing workshops and has had short stories and essays published. Along the way, she graduated from medical school and practiced full-time for six years; she is now a member of the academic/research faculty at Boston University Medical School.

aunt Helen sees a ghost

Laurie Douglas
4/23/2008

Five months ago my husband and I moved from Manhattan to Queens to take care of his 84-year-old aunt, who has Alzheimer's. Although she can't cook, shop, or manage her money anymore, Helen is remarkably functional in her own home. She's lived here almost forty years, more than half of them alone, as a widow.

Nothing has changed—the furniture, the bric-a-brac, even the refrigerator magnets—since my husband was a child. Neither has Helen's daily routine. She spends the day on autopilot, brewing cups of weak Lipton tea loaded with half-and-half, washing tiny machine-loads of hankies and hand towels, and making her way through the house at dusk, flicking on plug-in nightlights along the way. It's the perfect setup for someone with dementia; she can do a lot without having to think.

Ironically, Helen hates this house, curses it daily. It's a constant reminder of what she can no longer do, and she still feels responsible for maintaining it, even though we reassure her that we take care of it now.

A few days ago, she and I watched *That's Entertainment* (perfect, no plot). It was odd; every time a different movie star came on screen, she asked if the person were dead.

Helen: That one's down in the ground now, right?

Laurie: Yep, he died a long time ago.

Helen: How far down is he?

Laurie: I'm not sure. Maybe twenty years.

Helen: Well . . . it sure would be nice if we could grab them and pull all of them back up and have them in this room with us. I feel so bad they're all gone. Some day I'll go down in the ground, too, and push my husband over. And that will be that. I wonder what it will be like . . . I wonder . . . .

Laurie: I like to think that when we die, we go out of our bodies and fly around for a while, that we can see everything and go everywhere. I think it will be nice.

Helen: Did you ever see that?

Laurie: What? Have I ever flown up in the air? I haven't, but some people can do it. My friend Teresa says she used to fly up out of her body into the corner of the room and then watch herself down below, sitting on the couch! Can you imagine?

Helen: A couple of days—I mean, a couple of weeks ago—I saw something like that.

Laurie: You went out of your body?!

Helen: Well, no. I was sitting here, with that on (*gestures to the TV*), and I thought I saw something standing right over there. It scared me. I wasn't sure. Was I sleeping? Was it in my head? But I did see something.

Laurie: You think you saw a ghost? Wow. Did you know who it was?

Helen: No, it wasn't anyone I knew.

Laurie: What did it look like?

Helen: I can't remember. I am so stupid, it's this stupid head (*she taps her forehead with her middle finger*).

Laurie: You're not stupid, we all forget things. Maybe it'll pop back into your head in a day or so.

Helen: I'm not sure about that. But I saw something. It scared me. I didn't look over at it, and I tried really hard not to think of it.

Laurie: If it happens again, or if you're ever scared about anything, come upstairs and knock on our door. Even in the middle of the night. I'll wake up. I'll go down and look. If it's a ghost, I really want to see it! (*We both laugh.*)

Helen: I don't know what it was about. Maybe I imagined it.

Laurie: You could have been dreaming and just thought you were awake. Or you could've seen something that wasn't there, it's called hallucinating. It's nothing to worry about. Why were you scared? Did whatever it was seem mean or angry?

Helen: Not really . . . *(long pause)* I thought maybe I was going to go in the ground.

Laurie: Oh . . . Did you feel sick?

Helen: No, I was just sitting here watching with the lights on.

Laurie: Wow. TV and lights on and everything. Well, I don't know what you saw. But the good thing is that you're still here! *(We both laugh.)*

Helen: Yes ma'am! I'm here, and everyone else is gone. Eighty-four years. Too much!

Laurie: I tell you what: when you die, if you get to fly all around, will you come back and see me?

Helen: No way! I'm getting OUTTA this friggin' house!

—————————————

About the author: *Laurie Douglas is art director of* Pulse—voices from the heart of medicine. *Six months after this story was written, Aunt Helen moved to a studio apartment on the dementia-care floor of an assisted-living facility. She says she likes it there because she doesn't have to "work" anymore. Helen turned 87 in February 2009.*

Redesigning the practice of medicine

Pamela Mitchell
5/7/2008

what if we went slowly   thoughtfully   about the business of healing
what if I bowed   to you and you to me   before we touched aching bodies
what if we said   out loud   this   is sacred work   might I be made   worthy
what if I blessed your hands   and you mine   before we began
repairing   delivering   dressing   listening to
broken bodies   hungry souls

would we then return   to the place   where so long ago   we felt called
where we knew for sure that   we did indeed   have hearts
hearts that beat confidently   full   of ambition
hearts that were courageous   enough to break
again   and again   and again
hearts that were not afraid   to weep

at the sheer beauty of   fulminating organ
the raw pain   of splintered fracture
the howling loss   of bodily movement

what if we were unafraid to weep   at the joy   of newborns crowning
or the resurrection   of hearts expired

what if we were unafraid   to say   I do not know the answer
and welcomed Humility   into our practice
what if we sat down with Her   said a blessing
and quietly contemplated
the Mystery

About the poet: A nurse for thirty years, Pam Mitchell RN MFA currently enjoys nursing in mental health. She was anthologized in Intensive Care *(University of Iowa Press, 2003) and has been published in other literary venues.*

About the poem: "Redesigning the Practice of Medicine *was born in a moment of deep grief and frustration. I was reflecting upon the many years I'd spent in my profession and longing for the days when I'd had more time with patients. I remembered a sense of collegiality and a more humane approach to providing care. Those were rare and cherished times that I continue to long for and seek out. In writing this poem, I began to realize a great deal about the privilege granted by being a nurse. When I realized how many bodies I had held, rocked, covered and touched, I began to shudder with a sense of sheer awe."*

My War Story

Marc Tumerman
5/16/2008

My practice is in a small rural Wisconsin town just down the road from a large military base. I see soldiers pretty regularly these days; they stay here for several weeks of pre-deployment training before shipping off to Iraq. They come from all over the country—men and women of various ages, some single, some married and with families. Their health-care needs aren't too different from those of my civilian patients: maternity care, chronic illness management and the usual scrapes and bruises. I like having them on my schedule; their Boston accents and Georgia drawls make a pleasant change from my neighbors' familiar, made-for-radio Midwestern monotone.

I don't dwell much on what these soldiers do for a living. I do my best to take care of their needs and move on to the next patient. Once in a while, though, I run into one who sticks in my head at night as I lie in bed trying to make sense of the day.

Captain America is one of these patients. Sitting on my exam table, this 29-year-old man looks like a cross between G.I. Joe and the Terminator, his well-sculpted V-frame a walking advertisement for the U.S. military. He is soft-spoken and polite, concluding his answers to my questions with "sir." We mere mortals admire guys like this; they make us feel stronger and manlier by association. He's the kind of guy I would like to join for a day of fishing, smoking cigars and swapping tales.

He tells me that he's recently returned from two tours of duty in Iraq. Prior to that, he served in Afghanistan. As a captain, he led troops in clearing city neighborhoods of "insurgents." He's the guy you see on television, rifle in hand, breaking down doors.

Since returning from his last tour, a year ago, he has not been himself.

"I just feel whipped. I ache all over, and I'm tired all the time—no stamina. I get short of breath, and my chest aches just walking up a hill. I can't even sleep at night, doc."

He used to run six miles in under forty minutes, but now has trouble completing one. "Hell, you wouldn't believe the stuff I used to do." I can tell he wants me to know how tough he is, and that he's not looking for sympathy or a ticket to early retirement.

"Patch me up and send me back," he tells me.

As I listen to his story, I sift my memory for any reference to Gulf War syndrome. Was it real? What did the government's final report conclude? My gut tells me that the captain is depressed and possibly suffering from post-traumatic stress disorder. But I can't exclude the possibility of a toxic exposure to an as-yet-unidentified Agent X. How would the captain accept a diagnosis of depression? Would it offend this embodiment of strength?

He tells me that his last tour of duty was very stressful and left him disappointed and confused. Proud of what he'd accomplished during his first tour, he felt that what he'd seen this last time was unprofessional and reflected badly on our military and our country. "Unprofessional." Now there's an interesting choice of words.

I hesitate—afraid to ask for details. Despite my antipathy to this war, I still want to believe in my country. Hearing a first-hand account of the horrors of war, the inevitable mishaps and even the intentional and inherently human evils that occur, would force me out of the comfort of my insulated world. And yet I don't want to be complacent—a passive co-conspirator.

A series of lab tests, a chest x-ray, pulmonary function tests, electrocardiogram and a cardiac stress test reveal no clear explanation for this man's symptoms. The diagnosis of depression weighs heavy on my mind.

When he returns the following week, I admit that I've found nothing concrete to explain his dwindling strength: no kryptonite here. This should be good news, right?

He accepts a trial treatment with antidepressants. Within three weeks he's remarkably better. "I almost feel like my old self, doc!" But I can see that he's still troubled.

"Can depression really explain the way I was feeling?"

He confesses that he's questioning his role in this war and his career in the military. He doesn't think he can do another tour and is considering a desk job here in the

States. This bothers him because he was good at what he did, and the military needs experienced captains.

I feel troubled as well. It's quite possible that he suffered some physical injury in Iraq. I know that he's been dealing with depression and PTSD, but I still can't be sure that an Agent X didn't trigger his condition. I also don't know how well the military will deal with him or with the many other soldiers who return with significant psychiatric disorders after their Iraqi experiences.

We talk awhile, and I ask him to stay on his medications and to see me back in one month. He agrees; we shake hands.

I never see the captain again. Perhaps he shipped out for his fourth tour. Maybe he retired early. I try to contact him, but without success. Like I said, some patients just stick in my mind.

I like and respect this man of steel. I am awed by what he had to endure and sacrifice in Iraq. My feelings about this war do not make him any less of a hero, any less deserving of my admiration and affection or of the best medical care possible.

And yet, I'm left feeling unsettled. This man's name and face remain etched in my mind. He's but one of the thousands of young men and women left to carry the scars of this ill-conceived, needless war. I feel angry at our government for perpetuating it—and ashamed at my passivity as my young patients continue to ship out. My mind keeps circling back to a single thought: damn it, he should not have been there.

About the author: *Marc Tumerman MD has been a family physician practicing in Wisconsin for more than twenty-five years, during which time he has held various leadership roles involving practice management and quality improvement. "Like many, I have chosen to write about some of my more meaningful patient relationships because it's become clear that it is these relationships that give meaning and fullness to my life. In addition, writing serves as a way to help me deal with some of the frustrations and limitations that life places on us at work and at home."*

Mothers and Meaning

John G. Scott
5/23/2008

"Dr. Scott, this is Dr. Font." The call came from my mother's cardiologist as I was about to see my first patient of the morning. "Your mother is worse. You'd better come as soon as you can. I don't think she'll survive the day." Those blunt words shattered my denial: I had convinced myself that it was possible to fix the cumulative, lifelong damage wreaked on my mother's heart by her atrial septal defect, a congenital condition.

I thought back to the time, weeks earlier, when I'd gone to visit my parents. The vibrant, life-loving, intellectually engaged woman I knew so well was beaten down by her illness. Pain clouded her eyes and lined her face. I could see the bony outlines of her hips underneath her clothes.

I had sat up with her all night, feeling her racing pulse and holding her hand as she struggled to master her terror. Eyes closed, she repeated over and over, "Lord, give me strength. Lord, give me strength. Lord, give me strength." By morning, I felt exhausted—and ashamed to realize that my eighty-four-year-old father had been doing this for weeks. My medical objectivity vanished: all that mattered was to get my mother to the best doctors I could find. I chartered a plane to take her to a hospital in San Antonio, where my sister lives. As we rolled my mother's wheelchair across the threshold, she looked around at the house where she had raised three children and lived for fifty-three years with my father. "I guess this is the last time I'll ever see this place," she said.

"Don't be silly," I said, ignoring my own feelings of premonition. "We'll have you back to normal in a few weeks."

At the San Antonio hospital, that temple of medical technology, I felt sure that my mother's pain would be controlled, her heart fixed and her emaciated body nourished. The cardiologist there harbored no such illusions. He took me aside. "I'm not sure there's much we can do for your mother. I think you need to think about arranging for hospice care."

"Oh no," the child in me thought. "I can't do without my protector, my mentor, my confidant; not here, not now, not yet."

Over the next three weeks, I focused all of my energy on my mother's nutrition, convincing myself that if I could get her to gain weight, then her heart would function better too. My sister and father deferred to me, the family doctor, about treatment decisions. So I became the nutrition Nazi.

"You've got to eat, mother."

One bite, then a shake of her head. "I just can't do it."

"You're not trying hard enough!"

"I *am* trying!"

Unmoved by her tears, I convinced her internist to try intravenous feeding through a tube placed in a large vein in her chest. By morning, my mother was struggling for breath: her heart was too weak to handle the extra fluid. She couldn't talk, but I could see the fear in her eyes. Undaunted, I convinced her to have a feeding tube inserted in her nose. After one day, she begged me to remove it. "I can't stand this. Please, please take it out."

Still determined to feed her back to health, I pushed for placement of a PEG tube—a feeding tube surgically inserted into the stomach through the abdominal wall. Once again, her physicians honored my request, and my mother reluctantly acquiesced. The circulation to her intestine was so poor, though, that she couldn't absorb the feedings. Not only was the resulting alternating diarrhea and constipation painful, but having to wear a diaper and being constantly soiled was the greatest indignity of all for this proud and modest woman.

After two weeks of this, the torment ended. One morning she regurgitated the PEG tube feeding, aspirated it into her lungs and slipped into a coma. She died peacefully with her family at her bedside.

Thinking back, I see now that my medical knowledge increased my mother's suffering at the end of her life. Why did I act as I did? As a family physician, I should have known better, but I behaved like many family members: I kept trying "one more thing," only to find that, in striving to save my mother's life, I caused her more pain and robbed her of the chance to find acceptance and meaning in facing her death.

Reflecting on this has painfully reaffirmed for me that health is more than a well-functioning body-machine; it is the dynamic process of making meaning of both life and death. We must learn how to be masters of, rather than be mastered by, our technology, so that our science serves the soul as well as the body.

Our mothers demand no less.

_____

About the author: John Scott MD PhD is an assistant professor of family medicine at Robert Wood Johnson Medical School in New Brunswick, New Jersey. Intending to be a pediatric neurologist, he received his MD and PhD from the Duke University Medical Scientist Training Program, but took a detour into family medicine. After completing a family medicine residency at the Medical University of South Carolina, he was a family doctor in rural Arkansas for twenty-one years. In yet another detour, he moved to New Jersey to learn qualitative research methods and now spends most of his time studying healing relationships between doctors and patients. His wife, Vicki, works with middle-school language arts teachers in the South Bronx. John has three grown (sort of) children who are, among other things, a medical anthropologist, a banker and a philosopher.

A Certain Anesthesia

Arthur Ginsberg
5/30/2008

Exhaustion sets in by day's end
when the old Pakistani woman
hobbles into my office.
Raccoon eyes underscore the pain
she feels in her left leg. More cavalier
than a Hippocratic disciple should be,
I pull up her djellaba* to expose
the dark, tumescent flesh of her calf
monogrammed by serpiginous veins.
I am too aggressive with the needles
that search for the source
of the white-hot poker lancinating
from ankle to groin, muscular infidelity.

She is stoic,
so well schooled in cruelty
that even I pretend not to see
the slight jiggle of her jaw, enough
to tell me I have crossed the border
of disrespect. Apocryphal as it may be,

this is what I have to give
at the end of the day, a certain anesthesia
for the provenance of pain, how
she stands after it is all over,
rearranges her covering, and leaves me
speechless with the tent of her hands.

* pronounced je-lab': A long, hooded garment with full sleeves, worn especially in Muslim
countries.

About the poet: *Arthur Ginsberg MD is a neurologist and poet based in Seattle. He has studied poetry at the University of Washington and at Squaw Valley with Galway Kinnell, Sharon Olds and Lucille Clifton. Recent work appears in the anthologies* Blood and Bone *and* Primary Care, *both from the University of Iowa Press. He was awarded the William Stafford prize in 2003.*

The pencil Man of western Boulevard

Paula Lyons
6/6/2008

His history was Dickensian. As a little boy, born with an IQ of about 80 and a wandersome nature, he'd toppled onto the train tracks and gotten run over. How he didn't die is a mystery—this was more than fifty years ago, and he lost both legs up to his hips—but live he did.

I met him in the hospital, where he'd had surgery on the pressure sores that came from long hours perched in a wheelchair. When I asked him to roll over so I could see, he hoisted his whole body (200 pounds without legs!) out of the bed via the orthopedic trapeze. His arms were massively strong, his disposition was sweet, and he spoke and behaved like a well-mannered six-year-old. "My name is Andy," he told me. "I like you."

At the nursing station, the charge nurse teased, "So now you've met the Pencil Man of Western Boulevard." That was how the folks of Baltimore knew him—I was caring for a minor celebrity! Every day except Sunday, Andy sat in his wheelchair on the sunny corner of Western and Eastham, next to a leafy park, selling pencils and chatting with passersby. It was not a bad life, by his account. On Sundays, he told me with secret glee, his brother let him drive his brother's truck in the deserted, furthermost parking lot of the mall. From what I could understand, Andy took the wheel and his brother sat close beside him and worked the pedals.

His brother, also impressively muscled, and resolutely taciturn, looked as if he'd never had a lick of fun in his whole life. It tickled me to think of them careening about the lot. Did they laugh together? I imagined these sixty-year-old men, boys again for a short time, at dusk out behind Penney's.

As an adult, Andy had developed type 2 diabetes, which mystified him with its blood-sugar-tracking requirements ("Too many numbers, Dr. Lyons!"). He also had cirrhosis of unknown cause—he didn't drink, and tests for viral hepatitis, Wilson's disease and hemachromatosis were all negative.

Andy lived alone in a tiny apartment; his brother and sister looked in on him. After his surgery, a visiting nurse and aide visited three times a week to help him change his dressings (he was afraid of blood) and to bathe.

Despite this additional care, he began to show up in my clinic nearly every week with some small complaint: shoulder pain that couldn't be reproduced in the office; a stomachache (now gone); a sore in his mouth. I was mystified: the prior records showed that he came rarely, even to planned appointments. His cirrhosis was stable, his blood sugars weren't too bad, he didn't seem depressed. What was going on? I called his brother.

"Nah, he seems fine to me, Doc."

At each appointment, Andy listened happily to my advice, smiled charmingly, his bad teeth showing, and accepted willingly whatever salve, pill or cream I offered. I commented on this at the clinic desk and saw the nurses' smiles and covert glances.

"What?" I asked suspiciously. "What do you know that I don't?"

"Paula, you are an idiot," said Becky, our gum-cracking nursing tech. "The man is in love with you."

When I'd been a resident, one of our best attending physicians had said, "You'll never make a diagnosis unless you first think of it as a possibility." Becky was right— and I didn't know what to do. Annoyed, I found myself blushing when Andy and I were alone in the exam room. I decided that I *was* an idiot and carried on in a "professional" manner, though inwardly touched.

Lulled into complacency by Andy's stream of innocuous complaints, I felt startled and concerned when he came in with a new tremor in both arms. Feeling out of my depth, I involved Neurology, who had no answers either.

"Possibly a tiny basal ganglia stroke; did you rule out Wilson's disease? We can try some pharmacotherapy . . .."

The drugs made Andy feel bad, so he didn't take them, but the tremor was an increasing problem. Pencils fell from his grasp, he could no longer eat soup (his favorite), and he felt "wobbly" when transferring from wheelchair to bed.

With perfect bad timing, his pressure sores finally healed, and his visiting nurse and aide's services were terminated. I tried to get them back on the grounds of this new tremor ("Doesn't require skilled nursing care, Doctor") and that he needed help with finger-sticks ("Not if he's not on insulin, Doctor"). Finally I fudged, saying that I was worried that his liver disease might cause internal bleeding, and that he needed frequent blood tests drawn at home ("Is he truly housebound, Doctor?"). Nothing worked.

Some time later, with a sense of my worst fears being realized, I listened to his brother's gruff voice and watched him turn the brim of his hat over and over in his calloused hands as he described how Andy had fallen between the bed and the wheelchair when trying to transfer; he had lain there almost a day. Now Andy was in another hospital—a quirk of the EMS system—and "not doin' so well."

I went there after rounds. Relying on the happy anonymity of my white coat and stethoscope, I visited the ICU and reviewed his chart. Rhabdomyolysis (muscle breakdown), a heart attack, kidney failure . . . they also suspected a ruptured disk in his neck, as Andy's arms were now virtually paralyzed. An MRI was planned.

I let myself into his ICU cubicle.

"Andy." I leaned over the bed so that he could see me despite the hard collar on his neck.

"I'm scared," he whimpered. "I hurt. They want to put me in that tube."

I called his docs. They were understanding, and arranged for him to have an accessible MRI at a time when I could be there, as Andy had requested that I come along.

When the time came, he was apprehensive despite the Valium. The techs let me sit at the side of the arc. I stroked his hair. His breath was terrible.

I soothed him as I did my infant daughters: "*Shhh, shhh*, it's okay, I'm right here."

He giggled nervously, then slept. The MRI pictures added spinal-cord bruising to the list of Andy's woes.

I'd love to be able to report a happy ending to this story, but Andy died. His docs used every possible intervention to assuage his fear without prolonging the inevitable. To me, Andy's death was no less painful than that of any frightened child—for that is what he was, despite his massive biceps and mature frame. Coward that I am, I couldn't bring myself to attend his funeral, fearing that I might cry in public; but I did call his brother and write his sister a note.

I think of Andy often, see his grin and hear the cadence of his slow "Bal'more" speech. My life is richer for having known him. After all, not every doctor can claim that she once won the heart of the Pencil Man of Western Boulevard.

About the author: *Paula Lyons MD is a graduate of Emory University School of Medicine practicing family medicine just outside Baltimore, Maryland. Some of her other writings have appeared in* The Pharos *and* The Journal of Family Practice.

A Brush with the Beast

Paul Gross
6/13/2008

It all begins one Sunday morning when Mrs. Morris, a seventy-five-year-old retiree with a heart condition, trips on her way out of church. She falls flat on the sidewalk, can't get up, and ends up in our Bronx emergency room. A CT scan shows a pelvic fracture, and she's admitted to our inpatient team.

When I join the family medicine residents to see Mrs. Morris the following day, she can't get out of bed. She's got short, unruly white hair and a gee-whiz expression that charms us. "What a pain!" she says. Given how close she lives to the brink— terrible circulation has cost her one heart attack and several toe amputations—I'm impressed with her good cheer.

Things looks promising. Follow-up studies confirm that the fracture won't require surgery, and in the afternoon a physical therapist pilots her through a few wobbly steps.

The next morning we come to Mrs. Morris's room and find her peering at a novel. "I think it would be great fun to be a secret agent, don't you?" she says to me.

We make arrangements to transfer her to a rehabilitation facility, where therapy will get her walking again.

All goes smoothly until a hospital discharge planner hands me a slip of yellow paper. "Call this doctor," she says. "Insurance is denying the admission."

Uh-oh. I feel a sudden chill. A beast—Denial of Care—lurches over the horizon.

Looking glumly at the phone number, I recall a bout with the beast two days prior: puzzling over three different identification numbers on a patient's insurance card; navigating an automated telephone menu; waiting on hold; being told by a live person to call a different number; then being told at *that* number to try yet *another* number; and finally, being informed that neither my patient nor myself were in the insurance computer system.

This time, I'm in luck—sort of. The phone picks up right away, only it's not the doctor I want; it's someone else's voicemail. Did I dial right? I try again and get the same not-who-I-want message asking for the patient's insurance number, which of course I don't have.

Hanging up, I say a bad word. Then I go looking for Mrs. Morris's chart which, when I find it, doesn't seem to have her insurance information. I pause, frustrated; then someone interrupts me with a question about another patient.

Later that day, Meg, our social worker, comes over. "We've got a bed for Mrs. Morris, but her insurance is denying rehab. They say they're having trouble reading the therapist's note."

The beast again.

I don't picture it as a giant or troll. Rather, I imagine this maker of mayhem as a robot. Its iron torso shields a maze of electronic wires. Its taunting voice recites, "Your call is very important to us." Claim forms geyser from its metal fists and flutter around its blank face.

Armed with pens, telephones and determination, we all—health professionals and patients alike—leap to the challenge. The beast barely stirs. It's got all the time in the world.

Meg interrupts my reverie by grabbing a phone to locate the therapist with deficient penmanship. Failing that, she tries to wheedle another therapist into writing a note. Meanwhile, I find Mrs. Morris's insurance number, call the voicemail again and leave a message.

Time passes; the workday draws to a close.

Hospital day number three dawns. "You're still here!" I say to Mrs. Morris with attempted enthusiasm. "Well, the food's good," she says.

I leave another voicemail message.

That afternoon, I get a return call from a doctor with a soft, quavery voice. I wonder if she gets yelled at a lot. I sit down and take a deep breath.

"I understand that you're denying this admission," I say civilly.

"Well, according to the x-rays there wasn't anything requiring surgery, so it's not clear that the hospitalization was required."

Who, I wonder, would send a seventy-five-year-old cardiac patient home with a broken pelvis at 10:30 on a Sunday night?

"She was in pain," I say. "She's got heart disease. She couldn't walk." I forget to mention her missing toes.

"I'll pass that along," she says half-heartedly. "They'll take it into consideration. You can always appeal . . ." At the thought of another telephone safari, I feel my foot start to jiggle.

"*She couldn't walk,*" I repeat.

Hours later, I run into Meg. "Mrs. Morris is leaving!" she says. "They approved rehab—and the admission, too."

I'm pleased. After only a minor skirmish, the beast has clanked back to its lair. But I'm also annoyed. We've been giving Mrs. Morris excellent care. Why the hassle?

As a family physician and as a patient, I'm genuinely curious about this beast, Denial of Care. Mrs. Morris's story seems innocuous, but the same tale played out many times daily all over the country suggests something more profound at work.

How big is this beast? How many hours a day do we, as patients or health providers, grapple with it? How does this struggle affect the care we give and receive? On a deeper level, how does it square with our nation's spirit and soul?

And why doesn't it generate more notice? Have we simply come to accept it? Are we numb to its affronts?

Or is the opposite true: that each rebuff hits a raw nerve, producing cries too painful to voice—or too angry to listen to?

As *Pulse*'s editor, I hope that we can use one another's stories as yardsticks to take the beast's measure. I hope we can find plain, heartfelt words to describe disquieting fairy tales where giving and getting proper care demands a fight—and sometimes doesn't happen at all, despite our best efforts.

I hope, too, that our stories can illuminate and build on our strengths—our compassion, courage and resourcefulness—so that we can one day bring this beast to heel and our health care system back home to us.

About the author: *Paul Gross MD is editor-in-chief of* Pulse—voices from the heart of medicine.

summer

Reference Range

Veneta Masson
6/21/2008

Your tests show
the numbers 73, 90, 119 and 2.5,
the letter A,
the color yellow,
a straight line interrupted by a repeating pattern
of steeples and languid waves,
a gray asymmetrical oval
filled with fine white tracery,
35 seconds,
100 millimeters,
II.

I'm not sure what to make of these.
With the possible exception of II,
which like all Roman numerals
is subject to misinterpretation,
I see no cause for alarm.
I admit to a preference for low numbers,
the apothecary system over the metric
(my age, perhaps, and distrust of pure logic)
and the letter W,
though most of my colleagues favor
M.

I think you can be happy with yellow
and, based on my experience,
the fact that the straight line is punctuated.
Seconds, millimeters—I marvel at their finitude,
but this oval, so intricate, so light,
might well contain a universe.
Is it normal, you ask.
Normal's a shell game you seldom win.
Take my advice. Enjoy good health
not as your due but the blessing it is
like Spring, laughter,
death.

About the poet: *Veneta Masson RN is a nurse and poet living in Washington, DC. She has written three books of essays and poems, drawing on her experiences over twenty years as a family nurse practitioner and director of an inner-city clinic. Information about her poetry collection* Clinician's Guide to the Soul *is available at sagefemmepress.com.*

About the poem: *"Sometimes my muse takes the form of a curmudgeonly old physician who's weary of gold standards and unrealistic expectations about what medicine can offer. But he's also got a wry sense of humor and a useful perspective on health and illness. It's his voice that you hear in this poem."*

finding innisfree

Lawrence Dyche
6/27/2008

Roger looked up at me over the oxygen mask, his eyes drawn wide by the sores stretching his face. He lifted a hand for me to take.

"I'm glad you're here," Jen had said before I'd entered his room. "They've taken him off a lot of the medication. He's very lucid, but he's depressed and scared."

The previous fall, Roger and Jen had begun couples therapy with me. They were both thirty-two and had been together for ten years. Three years before they came to me, Roger had been diagnosed with leukemia. A bone-marrow transplant had left him cancer-free, but his prognosis was guarded. He and Jen argued frequently, his desire for independence clashing with her insistence on managing his care.

When they first visited my office, Roger shuffled in, bent and thin, on a walker. He wore a baseball cap, pulled low to shield his light-sensitive eyes. When he removed it, I saw that his face was covered with scabs, his bald head mottled in odd colors.

Jen spoke first, asking how much I knew of Roger's medical situation. I shared what I'd been told, being careful not to paint too negative a picture. Then Roger spoke. His calm, thoughtful voice provided a stark contrast to his physical appearance. He seemed remarkably free of resentment about his condition. As he described the ways in which leukemia was shrinking his world, he occasionally smiled faintly and absentmindedly stroked a missing eyebrow.

During our sessions, I learned that Roger had gained a reputation among his doctors as an inveterate fighter, and that neither he nor Jen seemed inclined to consider the very real possibility that he might not survive. I avoided challenging their denial—and soon fell into it myself, despite the fact that Roger couldn't seem to gain weight. Gradually, I fell in love with them as if they were my own children—not always the best move in my trade. Perhaps I felt awed by their courage; perhaps I still ached from the death of my estranged brother the year before.

Roger's hospitalizations grew more frequent and, as the April rains arrived, his individual therapist called to tell me that Roger's current hospital stay was likely to be his last. So I went to see Roger and Jen in the hospital. I felt the unnerving conviction that I needed to do something to help them prepare for Roger's dying.

Death is not a familiar to me. My parents died quickly and far away. I myself am hopelessly hypochondriacal; a new ache can throw me into a panic about my own mortality. I've read the literature on working with the dying, but it's always seemed too formulaic. I felt ill-equipped to help Roger and Jen that day.

The hospital was old and large and Byzantine. I wound my way through the long corridors to Roger's area. Jen greeted me at the doorway and asked me to see Roger alone.

I leaned over the bed, close above his oxygen mask. Straining to breathe, he told me that he was growing weary and that he didn't know if he could continue to fight. But each time he tried to tell Jen, the fear in her eyes stopped him.

I felt myself straining along with Roger's labored breaths. The very determination that drove Roger and Jen to battle his illness, and sometimes one another, seemed now to deny them the peace they so deserved. As the rain sighed at the window, a thought took shape in my mind. I touched Roger's gaunt shoulder.

"Life shouldn't only be about fighting, should it?" I asked.

Roger lay quiet for a minute, then asked me to bring Jen in. She sat down and began discussing his medications. I interrupted, telling her that Roger was having a hard time talking to her—that he was worried that she might not be able to go on without him.

"I can't even think about that, Roger, but I don't want to stop you from talking to me," she said.

"Jen, you've taken a lot from me—"

"Roger, I—" she began. Almost reflexively, I reached to stop her.

"Just listen," I said.

"Jen," he continued, "you are my soul."

With this, I left them together, found my way through the long corridors and stepped out into the pouring rain. Lines from Yeats' poem *The Lake Isle of Innisfree* were running through my mind:

> *And I shall have some peace there, for peace comes dropping slow,*
> *Dropping from the veils of the morning to where the cricket sings . . .*

Two days later, Jen called early in the morning to tell me that Roger had died peacefully the night before, with her beside him. Despite her grief, she thanked me profusely for the talk I'd had with Roger, saying that it had calmed him, helped him to reach a different place.

I fought the urge to say that I hadn't done anything—or at least that I hadn't known what I was doing.

Instead, I just listened.

About the author: *Lawrence (Larry) Dyche ACSW is a social worker who teaches primary-care residents at Albert Einstein College of Medicine. He has used narrative and poetry in his teaching and in personal reflection throughout his career.*

our town (chinese spoken)

Juan Qiu
7/11/2008

By the time Mrs. Zhang came to see me, her headache, left-sided weakness and facial numbness were two weeks old. Like many Chinese immigrants in this country, she'd hesitated to seek medical care because of language and cultural barriers and her apprehensiveness about Western medicine. In fact, she hadn't seen a physician in the ten years since she and her husband had come to America. Only after a friend told her about me, the sole Chinese primary-care physician in a small Pennsylvania town, did she and her husband come to see me.

Mr. and Mrs. Zhang struck me as a typical older Chinese couple. With smiles on their faces, they bowed repeatedly to everyone in my office. Mr. Zhang spoke English reasonably well, but Mrs. Zhang spoke only Chinese. She grasped my hands and kept telling me how grateful she was to be seen; after several moments, her husband had to gently remind her to let go of me.

Although Mrs. Zhang's other symptoms had resolved, her blood pressure was significantly elevated. Suspecting a stroke, I recommended a CT scan of her brain and medication for her hypertension. I also advised that she monitor her blood pressure at home and follow up with me in a couple of weeks. As I do with most of my Chinese patients, I wrote her instructions in a mixture of Chinese and English.

Seeing Mrs. Zhang reminded me of my own early experiences in this country. Shortly after I'd arrived, seventeen years ago, I'd had a bicycle accident and injured my ankle. Facing the same challenges as Mrs. Zhang, I didn't seek care until several months had passed. Unfortunately, this delay resulted in ankle pain that troubles me to this day.

A few days prior to the follow-up visit, Mr. Zhang called and requested his wife's CT-scan results. He hadn't been able to sleep, he said, for fear that she might have a brain tumor. "I don't want her to know the bad news," he said.

Suddenly I felt caught between two worlds colliding—worlds with different cultures, different expectations and different health-care delivery systems. In China, there is little concept of patient confidentiality. The family shields the patient from bad news, and the doctor joins in this "protecting" process. The patient is the last person to learn of an unfavorable diagnosis or prognosis and often never hears of it at all.

As a fellow Chinese, I understood and respected Mr. Zhang's wishes. As a physician practicing in the United States, however, I also had an ethical obligation to protect my patient's confidentiality.

When I told him that I couldn't divulge the information without his wife's consent, Mr. Zhang was shocked and bewildered. Nevertheless, after I explained about patient confidentiality, he agreed to provide a form, written by his wife in Chinese with an English translation, giving me permission to discuss her medical condition with him. Although not a typical informed consent, it served as a compromise solution in this difficult situation, and I was able to ease Mr. Zhang's worries—at least concerning cancer.

Mrs. Zhang's scan did show a hemorrhagic stroke. When they came to the office, I explained the cause of her stroke and the importance of treating her hypertension. Her home blood-pressure measurements had fluctuated significantly, and she admitted to taking her medication only every two or three days. "I feel fine. I have never taken Western medication before," she told me. The only reason she took the medicine at all, Mr. Zhang said, was to avoid disappointing me.

Although Mrs. Zhang's blood pressure was not optimal, it was better than before. I knew that it would take lots of education about her illness and about Western medicine before she would feel at ease with the treatment plan.

One of the nicest things about this story is that it has a happy ending—for the patient, the family and the physician. Over time, Mrs. Zhang has become comfortable taking Western medications. Her hypertension is under control, and she leads a full and active life with her husband. Recently I received a thank-you letter from Mr. and Mrs. Zhang: "We are grateful to have a Chinese doctor like you here in this small town."

It was written in Chinese *and* in English.

About the author: Juan Qiu MD PhD is an assistant professor and clinical faculty member in the Department of Family and Community Medicine, College of Medicine at Pennsylvania State University. "In addition to delivering patient care and teaching third- and fourth-year medical students, I participate in cultural-diversity awareness programs in the local medical community. I love caring for my patients, and I became interested in writing because I want to share what I have learned from them and be their advocate. I believe that both patients and providers need cultural-diversity education so that people of differing backgrounds can get equal access to quality medical care."

Echocardiography

Rachel Hadas
7/18/2008

One: secretarial computer screen:
appointments, cancellations. Two: machine

we're here for, registering your heart's each pump
with grainy images that throb and jump

in sync with the obscure interior.
Three: anticlimactic VCR

screen, a tiny, garish old cartoon
squawking and jerking in the darkened room.

Past these respective renderings of vision
we move next door. Here the examination

is palpable, is stethoscope to chest:
breath in, out, raise your arms, stand, squat, and rest.

I'm sitting, staring vaguely at the sky—
from the ninth floor, a pale blue vacancy.

What is a window but another frame
or screen through which to ponder—is it time

or space that peels this dull facade to show
the poverty of what we really know

despite the wealth of data we can see
via machines that pierce opacity?

Well, no more screens for one more year or two
Thank you and goodbye. It's time to go.

About the poet: Rachel Hadas is board of governors professor of English, Newark campus, Rutgers University. The latest of her many books of poems is The River of Forgetfulness *(David Robert, 2006);* Classics *(WordTech Communications), a volume of selected prose, was published in 2007. Her Web site is www.rachelhadas.com.*

first patient

Rick Flinders
7/25/2008

It was a quiet knock on my door that morning. So quiet, in fact, that I wondered if I was dreaming. Maybe if I went back to sleep it would go away.

Nope. There it was again: soft but persistent. This time I knew that it really was a knock, and it really was on the front door of my one-room cabin. What I didn't know was that I'd be hearing that knock for the rest of my life.

I got up, tired and rumpled, and pulled open the door. A young woman I'd never seen before stood there, barefoot and wearing the simple white linen dress of the *campesina* (as a woman who works the land is called in rural Paraguay). She was probably no more than sixteen, but in her eyes was the look of a mother, and something else: distress. In her arms she held an infant.

"*Xe memby o-hasy* (my baby's sick)," she said in her native Guarani.

I didn't understand a word, but I knew it wasn't good. I looked at her baby—face gray, eyes open, too sick to cry. What was I supposed to do?

Back then, I wasn't a doctor. Heck, I hadn't even taken any premed courses. I was just a liberal-arts major who'd "postponed graduation" from Berkeley "in order to get an education," as I explained to my incredulous father. Now I was the strange gringo (Peace Corps volunteer) living alongside a dirt road in the middle of the Paraguayan subtropics among a hundred or so peasant families, trying to help them literally hack a living from the jungle.

It was thirty miles to the nearest highway, 300 to the nearest hospital. This young mother had walked most of the night, from her home deeper in the jungle, to get to me. I was her last resort. She was out of options: there were no medicines and no doctors, and all the home remedies and the grandparents' ministrations obviously hadn't worked. Why not try the strange gringo?

"*Ja ha* (let's go)," I said, and motioned to my Honda 90 (Peace Corps issue) just outside the front door. I didn't know what else to do, but I couldn't do nothing. So I helped her onto the back of my motorcycle, where she clung, weeping, one arm clutching my waist and the other clutching her baby, and we headed for the crossroads where my little jungle road intersected the "highway." This route was just another dirt road, but it at least saw an occasional vehicle. One of these might transport her to the capital city, 300 miles away.

A half-hour later, almost within sight of the highway, the wailing in my ear suddenly changed. I knew what it meant. I stopped and got off. Then I held the young mother in my arms.

Speechlessly, in language that was neither English nor Guarani, I told her I was sorry.

We got back onto my motorcycle, turned around and headed back. For the next half-hour, I listened to the flood of a mother's grief—ceaseless, inconsolable, uncomprehending. The grief was hers and that of millions of mothers before her, across countries and cultures and time.

That sound, and her knock on my door that morning, has followed me through all the intervening years. It spoke to me when, after returning home, I changed my major from liberal arts to premed. It guided my choice to train in family medicine when I could have opted for other residencies. It is a gentle reminder when the frustrations of providing care in a seemingly deaf and broken healthcare system pile up. I sometimes wonder if I shouldn't have chosen something easier. But she always clears up my doubts.

I know now that she was my first patient, and will remain with me until the day I see my last. Even now, if I close my eyes, I can still hear her.

About the author: Rick Flinders MD has taught and practiced in Santa Rosa's Family Medicine Residency Program in Northern California for the past twenty-five years. "One of the great gifts of medical practice is what we learn, not just about medicine, but about life. I find writing hard, but well worth the effort, for what it teaches us and allows us to share. I try to encourage our residents to do the same." He can be reached at flinder@ sutterhealth.org.

once

David Goldblatt
8/1/2008

Movement disorders can be horrifying. Afflicted persons are solidified or contorted. They may flail so violently that a fork endangers their lives. As a beginning neurologist, I assumed that all such patients curse their fate. Once I got to know Brian, though, I realized that I could be wrong.

Brian and one of his brothers had inherited Wilson's disease, a rare, genetic movement disorder that had spared their eight siblings.

People who have Wilson's disease can't handle dietary copper properly. It accumulates in—and poisons—the kidneys, liver and brain. Avoiding foods rich in copper does not halt the progression of the disease, but it helps. If patients are also treated early and consistently with a drug such as penicillamine, which binds copper and aids in its excretion, they can expect to live a normal lifespan. If not treated, they die young.

Oscar, Brian's younger brother, was less affected than Brian in his movements and speech. He looked out for Brian in an unusual way: he punched, pushed and made fun of him. (Psychiatric disorders are common in the disease.) Oscar died in his twenties in a car accident. His spleen, swollen because of Wilson's-related liver disease, ruptured, and he bled to death internally.

After Oscar died, Brian spent some months in the county hospital, where a homeless man with a chronic illness could find care. Always, it seemed, he had a pretty student nurse at his side, and she was usually laughing. With his long, straight black hair, aquiline nose and lean, well-muscled body, he looked like—perhaps was—a Native American. Instead of showing the grace one might expect from someone with his looks, however, he moved stiffly. The harder he tried, the harder his anaconda muscles wrenched him back. Only sleep brought relief.

Speaking was especially difficult for Brian. It took him many seconds to begin to vocalize, and he often resorted to a letter board. Even then, his contrary musculature presented a challenge: his arm might snake toward the letter he wanted to touch but jerk away just as he was about to reach his goal. When he did try to speak, his tongue might protrude grotesquely. With great deliberateness, he would extend his index finger and thrust his tongue back into his mouth, then slowly and indistinctly articulate what he wanted to say. It was an exhausting experience, both for him and for the listener.

I was a member of an investigative team trying to treat the symptoms of Wilson's with various drugs used for Parkinson's disease. My assignment was to record Brian's status on videotape at regular intervals. Although treatment helped him, he was not always a compliant patient.

A tape we made in the eighth year of our association shows me pulling a blue packet of cigarette papers from Brian's shirt pocket and asking, "What's this?"

"Pay . . . pers," he says, with a slow, mischievous grin.

"What do you do with them?"

"They're for mari . . ." He haltingly continues: ". . . WAH . . . na."

"How often do you smoke it?"

The words come more freely: "Whenever I can get my hands on some."

Later in the session, I ask Brian about his favorite foods. He says that he loves Reese's Peanut Butter Cups.

"What's in them?" I ask.

"Peanut butter and chocolate"—two high-copper foodstuffs he knows he's not supposed to eat.

"Why would you eat something like that?"

"Because . . . I en . . . joy it!"

"But if you know it's bad for you . . .?"

Struggling to produce the words, but smiling serenely, he reminds me, "We . . . only . . . live . . . once."

About the author: David Goldblatt MD was a neurologist, writer, editor, potter, gentleman and avid slo-pitch softball player. A native of Cleveland, Ohio, he completed his medical degree at Case Western Reserve University in 1955 and his neurology residency at the New York Neurological Institute. After becoming chief of the neurology branch at the National Naval Medical Center in Bethesda, he conducted research at Johns Hopkins University, then spent thirty-one years at the University of Rochester as a professor of neurology and, later, as a professor of the medical humanities. His main medical interests were ALS, medical ethics, compassionate patient care and traumatic brain injury. David died of cancer at age seventy-seven on September 1, 2007.

physician's exasperation

Howard F. Stein
8/15/2008

We know so much about you—
Your blood, your urine, your internal organs.
We can see everything.
There is precious little that
Is not wrong with you medically.
Still, you do not listen to us.
You miss appointments;
You don't go to referrals we've made.
Do you defy us or merely not understand
How dire your condition is?
You could die at any time,
We have told you more than once.
Still, you muddle along as if all we know
Does not matter. Tell me, what
Is missing from our story?
Have we failed to impress upon you
The urgency of the hour? Speak to me.
I will listen now.

About the poet: *Howard Stein PhD, a psychoanalytic and medical anthropologist, is a professor in the Department of Family and Preventive Medicine at the University of Oklahoma Health Sciences Center in Oklahoma City, where he has taught for thirty years. A poet as well as a researcher and scholar, he has published five books of poetry, including* Theme and Variations *(Finishing Line Press, 2008). In 2006 he was nominated for Oklahoma Poet Laureate.*

About the poem: *"The search for control—real, imagined, wished-for—is at the unstated core of much of medical 'competence.' Not only are diseases often 'out of control,' but patients are likewise beyond physicians' control. In the face of repeated struggles to gain patient 'compliance' or 'adherence' to medical advice, and after engaging in 'patient education' for the umpteenth time, physicians wonder how they can possibly help the patient. Sometimes, a moment of grace arrives: The physician relinquishes the quest for control and enlists the patient's help in the form of storytelling. 'What is your story, your experience, from which I can learn how to help you?' the physician asks in many different ways. Sometimes a remedy for physician exasperation is deep, attentive listening."*

Losing Tyrek

John Harrington
8/22/2008

Tyrek's mother and I must have spoken for two hours in the Pediatric Intensive Care Unit, covering every topic but the one that was glaring at us: death. A fourteen-month-old child is not supposed to die—and even though I knew the situation was dire, I couldn't bring myself to face it. So I excused myself, sat down with her son's chart and stared blankly at it.

I first met Tyrek and his parents when he was just three months old. Tyrek had Down syndrome, clubbed feet and a large sternal scar on his chest from surgery to repair a complicated heart defect. Despite his bad luck, Tyrek's most impressive characteristic was his cheery disposition. His mother was a tall African-American woman with straightened hair and warm eyes that always appeared weary. Tyrek's father stood well over six feet, a sharp contrast to the "little man" he held in his arms.

I became Tyrek's pediatrician through a referral from a cardiologist who knew that I care for children with special health needs and that I happen to have a son with severe autism. Tyrek's parents and I bonded quickly, our conversations more animated and collaborative than the typical doctor-patient exchange. Tyrek always arrived at the office cradled in his father's massive arms and with at least one foot casted. I relished these visits because his parents were always so proud of Tyrek's accomplishments and always let me share my latest story about my own son, Sean.

Sean has difficulty communicating. Yet when we met Tyrek and his parents by chance at the neighborhood Staples, Sean wanted to touch Tyrek's cast. Carefully, Tyrek's mom explained that the foot wasn't straight, so the doctor had put it in a cast to fix it. My son nodded and said, "Good boy Tyrek!" as we all smiled approvingly.

Those smiles faded from my memory as I found myself back in the ICU.

Tyrek's mechanical heart valve had not been working properly, and the surgery to correct it was unsuccessful. I stood beside Tyrek's bed and stared at the monitors while his mother sat on a makeshift bed. I was convinced that he'd pull through. He'd already beaten most of the odds.

When I was a resident, the nursing staff and other residents would look to me to lighten a difficult moment with humor. Now, with Tyrek's mother, I mentioned a conversation my youngest daughter, Maya, had had with me about her older sister, Claire. She'd said, "If Claire can play the clarinet, how come I can't play the Maya-net?" Tyrek's mom smiled for a moment.

Even as she did so, something inside of me wanted to reach out, embrace her and tell her that I was sorry I could do nothing. Instead, I resisted it and went home for the weekend.

I came to regret that decision. Tyrek died a few hours later.

Even though I had left my twenty-four-hour pager, home phone and cell number with the parents and staff, no one contacted me when Tyrek passed away that Friday night.

Maybe his parents and the staff felt that I'd already said my goodbyes. Maybe they thought that I would be busy playing with my kids. Maybe they were worried that I would feel guilty or depressed that Tyrek didn't make it. Or maybe they didn't give it a second thought. I felt cheated—even disappointed—by the staff and by Tyrek's parents for not notifying me. But inside, I felt most upset at myself for not seizing the moment earlier when I'd had the chance.

Now I had to wrestle with closure. I felt all the remorse I hadn't expressed at Tyrek's passing. At the same time, I couldn't bring myself to go to the funeral or wake; instead, I sent a letter of condolence. It simply said, "My deepest sympathies, we will all miss Tyrek. Dr. H. and family."

I wish I could say that Tyrek's parents responded to my letter with some reassurance that they'd felt my last hours with them were important. I never heard from them, and I'm left to wonder why. I think of the words of the English writer Joseph Addison: "Friendship improves happiness, and abates misery, by doubling our joys, and dividing our grief." I feel painfully aware that I missed a special opportunity to let down my guard as a doctor and, by acknowledging the friendship I felt for Tyrek and his parents, to share our common grief and our humanity.

About the author: John Harrington MD is a board-certified general pediatrician and the father of Claire (fifteen), Sean (thirteen) and Maya (twelve). He is the director of the general academic pediatrics division at The Children's Hospital of The King's Daughters in Norfolk, VA. "Writing has always afforded me the chance to go back and replay moments in time where I was conflicted and perhaps emotionally exhausted as a physician. It provides an opportunity to regain perspective and insight on many different levels."

jeannie

Andrea Gordon
9/5/2008

"The person with the contractions gets to pick the channel," I reassure Jeannie, as she tries to talk me into watching *The X-Files*. It's not my favorite, but I'm just the moral support—oh, and the doctor.

When she first came to see me, eight months back, Jeannie already had a four-year-old boy and didn't think that there was much my little white nulliparous self could teach her about pregnancy. I'd offer her my book-learned advice about pregnancy or suggest sources of support, and she would listen patiently, then do what she wanted. She did show up for all her appointments, and she humored me at times: although she refused to stop smoking pot for her nausea, she cut down a little "to make you feel better."

Jeannie shared everything without embarrassment. Well-trained resident that I was, I asked her about bleeding or discomfort during sex. She said that it sometimes hurt when she was on top, "But he don't like havin' to be up there doin' all the work."

Now, two weeks before her due date, she's come into the office contracting. Sure that this is it, she's already arranged care for her son. We make the ten-minute pilgrimage to the hospital. I ask who she'll have with her during labor. Looking at me with one eyebrow raised, she replies, "You."

Oh. Okay.

So I sit with her, and we watch *Wheel of Fortune* and *The X-Files* and chat. I hadn't realized how important it is to her to have her own doctor. While completing the paperwork to be admitted, she'd informed me, "That nurse figured I was with the clinic. But I said, 'No, my *doctor* is Dr. Gordon.'" A little satisfied smile at defying the nurse's expectations.

The pigeonhole they've tried to squeeze Jeannie into pinches her, and she's not about to stand for it. As we sit there, she tells me about her previous labor. They'd said she couldn't have any pain medicine because she was too far along. "I grabbed that man by the tie and said, 'Give me some morphine.' And he did!" Wary of the world, she adds, "Who you gonna trust? If you're black, you can't trust the police. Can't nobody trust lawyers. So you gotta trust your doctor."

I try to express gratitude, but she brushes me off, changing the channel to a talk show.

After twenty hours of dwindling contractions, some sleep and then eighteen laps around the floor the next morning, we conclude that she is not in labor, having stopped dilating at three centimeters the night before. Jeannie and I leave for our respective homes, knowing that this is not farewell but au revoir.

Two nights later I'm awakened by a call from Katherine, one of my fellow residents.

"Your patient is here in labor, and she's wild. Get here as fast as you can!"

Barreling into the hospital room less than ten minutes later, I see Jeannie thrashing on the bed, wailing, "Pain! Pain!"

Katherine tells me that they have been unable to get an IV into her because she won't stop writhing.

"Jeannie," I implore, "you have to hold still so they can do this and give you medicine for the pain."

"I can't, I can't, I can't," she moans, tossing from side to side.

Some inner drill sergeant surfaces: I put my face over hers and bark "Jeannie!"

She freezes for a minute, then whispers, "What?"

"Have I ever lied to you?"

A pause, then: "No."

"Okay, so listen to me. You can do this."

A combination of commands and reassurance gets the IV placed, Stadol given, Jeannie calmed. I stay next to her, bullying as needed when she begins to push. The bizarre intensity of our connection doesn't occur to me until she asks for some ice. I begin to leave, but my supervising attending jumps up from the rocking chair, saying, "I'll get it. You stay here."

Jeannie has a baby girl, Keesha, and for the next four months brings her faithfully to see me. Then it's time for our last visit, because I will soon be graduating from residency.

Through the whole visit, Jeannie refuses to meet my eyes. She addresses her comments to Keesha: "You find a good doctor, and she just leaves."

I try my best behavioral-science phrases. "I know that you're upset I'm leaving . . ."

Jeannie will have none of it.

"Got to find a new doctor again," she tells Keesha.

I tell her which doctor will be seeing her and Keesha, but she keeps her gaze averted and finally leaves with Keesha in the carrier.

She doesn't even say goodbye.

As she walks down the hall I consider going after her to hug her, but realize that this is far too public a place, even if she might otherwise want me to do so. So I just watch her strong, straight back recede as she goes and think, "I love you too, Jeannie."

About the author: Andrea Gordon MD is on the faculty of the Tufts Family Medicine Residency Program at Cambridge Health Alliance in Malden, Massachusetts. "Although I wrote poetry in high school, I had stopped until my advisor in residency told me, 'You should write poetry.' That was enough to start me writing again. I feel privileged to be invited into people's lives and to hear their stories."

Antibodies

Shanna Germain
9/12/2008

At twenty, I started working the HIV
ward, midnight to morning. Left my husband
sleeping, mouth-open to the air, to
drive through the dark body of the city.

Every shift, the warning about infections.
Me sliding on booties, disposable
gown and gloves. Even through the mask,
you could smell decay, the way viruses

swept through bodies. I did what was needed:
held hands through double-gloves, took blood
or confessions when I could, told off-white lies
to thin cracked lips that knew the truth.

Once, a year or so into it, I stuck
myself, pointed red end of an IV needle
left in a lab coat pocket. So small a thing
it almost didn't hurt going in, only

leaving, small pop and smear of two bloods mingled.
I put the wound to my mouth and sucked before
I thought. Fear rising, rinsed my tongue with soap,
spit someone's dark blood into the white scrub sink,

then gave my own blood to one of the other nurses
to be tested. At dawn, I roused my husband awake
with my newly tainted tongue, let him slide bare
into me, as though nothing was between us.

I tell this all like it was an accident:
someone else's lab coat, a needle forgotten
in a white pocket, three seconds of married
passion so strong my lips did not say, at risk.

But no. This was after I caught the cliché
of my life: his red scrawl across receipts hidden
in a desk drawer, the smell of lilacs in
his sleeves, the cleaving across the bedsides.

The things we do in fear are the things we don't
say. Hidden and rampant as a hotel room stay
on a credit card, or a string of genes
in a coat of protein, destined to repeat.

About the poet: Shanna Germain claims the titles of leximaven, girl geek, wanderlust-er, avid walker and biker, tree kisser, knife licker, steak-maker, book-nerd and She Who Fears Ticks. Her work has appeared in places like Absinthe Literary Review, The American Journal of Nursing, Best American Erotica, Juked, Salon *and* Tipton Poetry Journal. *Visit her online at yearofthebooks.wordpress.com.*

About the poem: "This poem came about because I was thinking of all the things that we do to protect ourselves, not just in the medical field but in life. Not just healthwise, but also to protect our hearts, our souls. And how easily that can all be undone—by someone else's actions or by our own. And how we live with those repercussions after. Or don't."

confidential

Sandy Brown
9/19/2008

I was on medical admit, taking call for unassigned patients, when I was summoned to take care of a seventy-nine-year-old, mildly demented woman with a large pleural effusion. I decided to go over her chest x-ray with our radiologist.

"I don't know what's causing the effusion," I said. "That's why I ordered her scan."

"I can tell you what's causing it," John said. "She has a tumor in her chest."

"How do you know that?" I asked incredulously. "All I see is a white-out."

"She was an inpatient here six months ago," John said, pointing to an old film, "and she had a two-centimeter lesion then."

Mrs. Howell had been unable to tell me about her previous hospitalization, so I retrieved her medical record from the computer. Sure enough, she had been admitted after a fall, having sustained a pelvic fracture and a cerebral contusion. A routine chest film had been misread by the ER doctor and then apparently had been overlooked by the attending on call; he had neglected to read the radiologist's report as well. Now the patient was back, six months later, with a malignant pleural effusion.

What to do? Should I bring my colleague's blunder to the medicine committee meeting, which could lead to public humiliation for him, and possibly to bad blood between us? Or should I just inform him confidentially?

I also had to wrestle with another decision: whether or not to tell Mrs. Howell's family about the missed x-ray report. I felt conflicted, my professional conscientiousness butting heads with my empathy for a colleague who wasn't a bad physician but who, in this case, just hadn't been careful enough.

My thoughts squirreled round and round. Patients and their families deserve to know the truth, but in this case, what good would it do? The mistake had been made six months ago, and, given Mrs. Howell's mental status, I doubted that she would have been a candidate for aggressive therapy even then. Diagnosing her cancer six months earlier wouldn't have made any difference to her outcome, I told myself, and it would only have added to her family's distress . . . or was this just a rationalization? Whatever my decision, I knew I couldn't feel good about it.

In the end, I opted not to tell.

The next day, I placed a copy of my colleague's original discharge summary in his box, along with the old x-ray report, the current CT report and a brief note, and waited for his response. Several days later, I ran into him while making rounds. After thanking me and expressing his concern for Mrs. Howell, he wondered aloud, a bit feebly, why the radiologist hadn't personally notified him about the tumor.

I felt for him. Fundamentally, we all have feet of clay; sooner or later, we all miss a big one. If we don't learn from our mistakes and use those lessons to become better physicians, then no one really benefits.

Since I always beat myself up over bad outcomes, I vowed to be even more vigilant. I knew how uncomfortable I'd felt telling my colleague about his mistake; I didn't ever want to put a colleague in the position of having to tell me about mine.

About the author: Sandy Brown MD practices family and preventive medicine in Fort Bragg, CA. For more than six years he wrote the column "Practice Diary" for the American Academy of Family Physicians (www.aafp.org). He now writes the "Family Medicine Practice Diary" for Medscape Family Medicine (www.medscape.com), as well as facilitating the site's family medicine and internal medicine discussion boards. His diaries have been translated into Chinese. When not writing or seeing patients, he enjoys dirt- and mountain-bike riding and counseling premedical students about how to get into medical school.

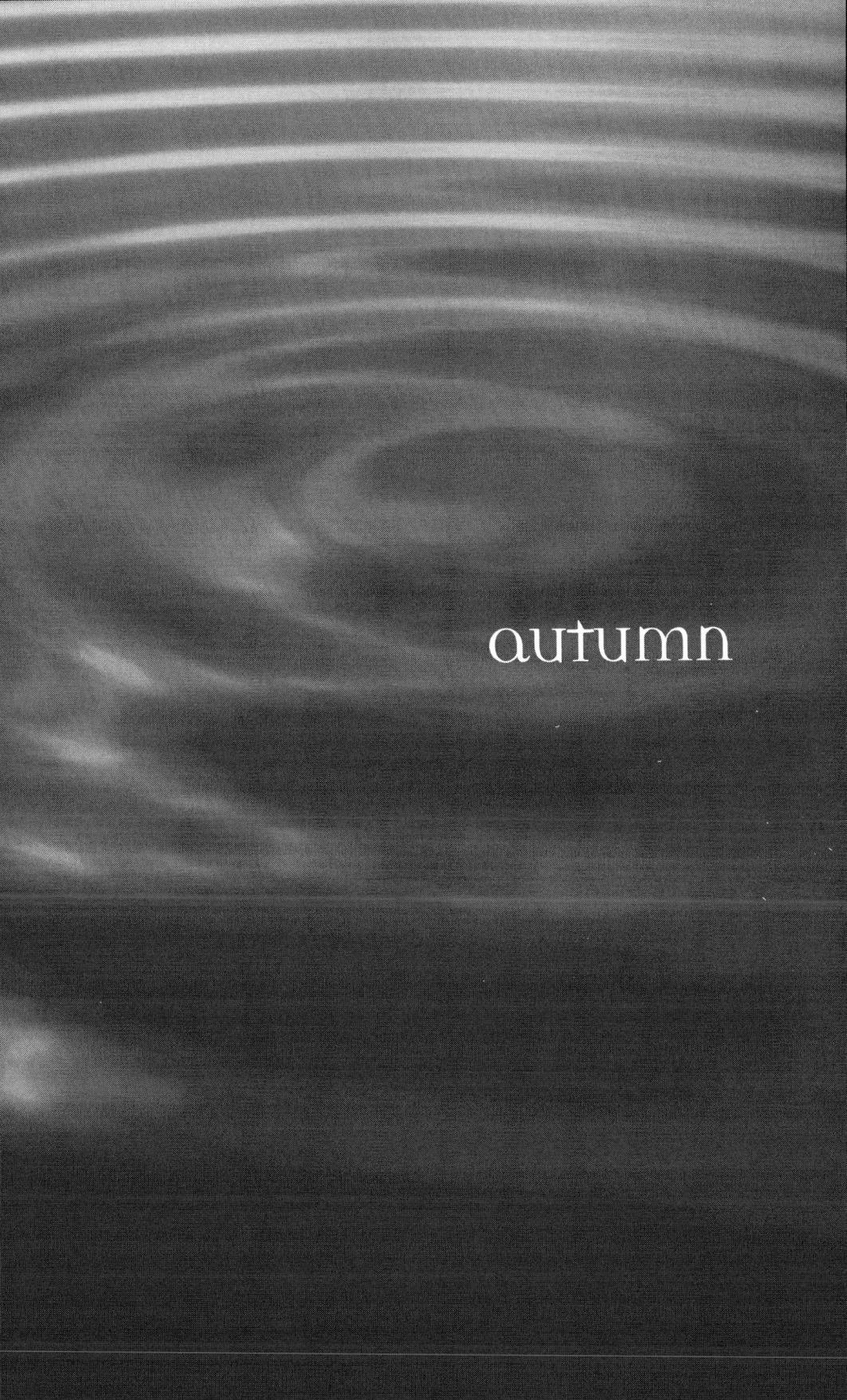

autumn

in the nick of time

Barry Thompson
9/26/2008

When the ringing woke me at 3:00 a.m., I hoped that it was my alarm clock. For a neurologist on call, middle-of-the-night phone calls mean trouble; as a rule, you don't get awakened at that hour unless it's something really serious.

At 6:00 p.m. the prior evening, a young man had shown up in the ER of one of our satellite hospitals with a severe headache. He'd been diagnosed with a tension headache and discharged with a prescription for acetaminophen with codeine. No imaging studies had been done.

Nine hours later, the patient presented to the ER at our main hospital. He was no longer fully alert, the ER doc told me. I told him to get an immediate CT scan of the head. I was out of bed and through the door in an instant, worrying about this young, otherwise healthy man with a severe headache and reduced alertness. It's amazing how fast you can drive in the dead of night when you're nervous that a life may hang in the balance.

I parked in my usual spot, right by the ER entrance, and ran inside. The nurse told me that the patient had been sent upstairs to get his CT. I dashed to the elevators and got to the CT suite in just a couple of minutes. By now I was running on adrenaline; as I swung the door open, I could feel my heart thumping in my chest.

Again, my timing was off; the patient now was on his way down to the ICU. I couldn't believe I'd missed him again. Luckily, his films were lying on the counter, and I slapped them up on the viewbox. When I saw what was on those films, my heart really started to pound. They showed a massive enlargement of the ventricles (fluid-filled cavities, normally quite small) inside his brain. The resulting increased pressure inside this young man's skull explained his headache and grogginess. I ran even faster down the stairs to the ICU, where I finally caught up with him.

To my surprise, he was still on the gurney, just as the transport people had left him. He was unconscious, his ER chart resting on his chest. Apparently, the nurses were in the middle of changing shift; no one there had even taken a look at him. He was just lying there, unattended. I couldn't believe what was happening; it was as if I were in the middle of some horrible dream.

After a few seconds' assessment, I realized that he was in the process of herniating: The increased pressure inside his head was pushing his brain down through the opening at the base of the skull, through which the brain and spinal cord connect. His left pupil was widely dilated and unresponsive to light, and he showed signs of damage to the motor pathways controlling his left side. Unless I acted immediately, he could be dead in a very short time.

I shouted to the nurses that he was herniating, which really got their attention. I told them to immediately give him a large intravenous dose of mannitol, a powerful diuretic.

Within seconds, as I anxiously watched over him, his pupil shrank back down to normal size. It was working!

After only another minute or two (or so it seemed; I was so amazed and overjoyed that it was hard for me to judge), he woke up! My patient, who had been on the brink of death just moments before, was now alert: He knew his name and where he was, and he could move all four limbs. I felt euphoric.

Walking on air, I approached the small room by the ICU where his mother and father were anxiously waiting. From their expressions, I could tell that they expected the worst. As I delivered the hopeful news, I fully realized the enormity of what had taken place: Had circumstances been just slightly different, I would have been informing them instead of their son's death.

Even now, after all these years, my eyes mist over when I recall that night. If I had missed just one more traffic light, or lingered in bed just a couple of minutes longer, or if there had been no parking spot right by the ER entrance, I believe that my patient would have died. (His symptoms, it turned out, were due to a noncancerous tumor inside one of his ventricles; following a successful operation, he made a full recovery.)

On that night so long ago, it seemed to me that some higher power, or fate if you will, placed me at that young man's bedside at exactly the right time. It seems a bit fantastic to me now, but back then it made perfect sense. I'm no longer a strong believer in fate, but when I relive that night in my mind, a powerfully spiritual feeling still comes over me.

I never again found myself in a situation in which my split-second actions at a precise moment in space and time allowed me to save another's life. Every time I think about that night, I thank God that I was lucky enough to have done just that.

About the author: Barry Thompson MD is a graduate of the University of Southern California School of Medicine. After engaging in the private practice of neurology for fourteen years, he left medicine in the late 1990s to become first a ballet photographer and then a psychotherapist. He lives with his wife and two children in the Pacific Northwest.

RX

Veneta Masson
10/3/2008

Politicians . . . were quick to rise to the defense
of a particularly vulnerable population. As a group,
dual-eligibles [Medicare-Medicaid] have incomes below
the poverty rate . . . and take an average of 15 medications a day.

Washington Post
January 14, 2006

This is how it works:
as wealth trickles down
to the poor and old
it turns into pills.

So M and S, their slender portfolios
long since depleted, can still
compete for bragging rights.
I take twenty a day, says M.
Ha! counters S, *I take so many*
they had to put in a port.

G presides over the corporate enterprise,
his specialty, mergers and acquisitions.
With combined assets (his own and his wife's)
filling two cupboards, he allocates resources,
tracks inventory, restocks
from Canada and Wal-Mart.

K can still indulge herself.
I'll start with one of the pale pink ones,
she tells the striped tabby,
but I might decide I need two or three.
I'll wait a while and see how I feel.
Maybe the purple would do me more good.

Honor is served.
Wealth is transferred.
The old have their pills.
And their health?
That's another story.

About the poet: *Veneta Masson RN is a nurse and poet living in Washington, DC. She has written three books of essays and poems, drawing on her experiences over twenty years as a family nurse practitioner and director of an inner-city clinic. Information about her poetry collection* Clinician's Guide to the Soul *is available at www.sagefemmepress.com.*

About the poem: *"When I first read the article in the* Washington Post *from which I took the epigraph for this poem, my mind flooded with memories of all the elders I've cared for over the years and what role their pills played in their lives. Talk about the placebo effect! It applies not just to the patient whose medication fills various roles, but to the professional who prescribes them and to the society which manufactures and pays for them."*

carmen's story

Carmen Diaz
10/10/2008

I used to be a shy woman who didn't like the spotlight and never did any public speaking. Ovarian cancer has changed all that. Now I look for opportunities to tell my story.

I am a sixty-two-year-old, Puerto Rican-born, New York-raised mother of two. I was diagnosed with ovarian cancer in 2004. But for more than a year before that, my symptoms weren't recognized.

In January 2003, I started to suffer from abdominal discomfort, back pain, indigestion and heartburn. My primary-care physician told me to change my diet and prescribed medication for my indigestion. After weeks with no improvement, I went to a gastroenterologist, who diagnosed gallstones. In March, I had gallbladder surgery.

Most people go back to work within ten days, but it took me a month. My fatigue, heartburn and stomach cramps, I was told, were probably a result of the surgery. Over the following months, I kept returning to my primary-care doctor, who prescribed antacids. Eventually, fearing that he'd brand me a hypochondriac, I stopped going.

That fall, during a routine gynecological check-up, I told my ob-gyn that I was feeling pelvic pressure and a burning sensation in my bladder. My pelvic exam and Pap smear revealed no abnormalities; she told me I had a urinary-tract infection and prescribed antibiotics.

By early 2004, I was having trouble eating: even after small meals, I felt full and bloated, and my stomach swelled. Family members began to ask jokingly if I were pregnant.

All my life, I'd been an avid tennis player and skier and exercised regularly. Now, fatigue and shortness of breath forced me to cut back on my workouts. My primary-care physician ordered a stress test, electrocardiogram and blood tests, which showed that I was anemic, so I took iron pills and began to feel better.

I hired a personal trainer to concentrate on abdominal exercises. After several weeks, though, I realized that no amount of training was going reduce my stomach. That April, determined to get my flat stomach back, I had a tummy tuck.

A few weeks later, the right side of my abdomen began to bulge. "It's probably a hematoma—residual blood," my plastic surgeon said, but he also ordered a CT scan and a blood test for CA125, a tumor marker.

The results were shocking: my abdomen was filled with fluid, and my CA125 was sky-high.

My plastic surgeon delivered the news: I had stage IIIC ovarian cancer that had metastasized to my pelvis, lymph nodes, bowel and liver. I was so stunned, I can barely remember a thing he said.

He also informed my primary-care doctor, whom I'd known for fifteen years. When I went to see him the next day, he was devastated. "I don't know how I'm going to talk to Carmen about this," he'd told his wife.

We spent a long time discussing the cancer. Reviewing my healthy lifestyle, he told me, "You did everything you were supposed to do." And he had already made an appointment for me to see a wonderful surgeon that very afternoon, so I couldn't be angry with him.

I do feel angry at my gynecologist, though. When I'd told her that I was having a tummy tuck because of my distended belly, she'd never mentioned the possibility of ovarian cancer; she'd only commented, "The next time I see you, you're going to have a nice, flat stomach." And when I told her about the cancer diagnosis, she only said that ovarian cancer is very hard to detect.

She made me feel that there was nothing anyone could have done, but I don't believe that. I feel so mad that I was misdiagnosed so many times. If I'd known about the symptoms of ovarian cancer, I could have gotten help earlier.

A month after being diagnosed, I had a total hysterectomy with debulking, followed by six rounds of Taxol and Carboplatin. Eight months later, a second-look surgery revealed more cancer cells. Cisplatin, delivered directly into my abdominal cavity, made me so ill that I had to be hospitalized for ten days. I went into remission for ten months.

Then, in April of 2006, more than a year after my hysterectomy, my pelvic pain started again. After negative MRI and PET scans, the doctor said that the pain might be caused by adhesions.

In June, during a procedure to remove them, one of my intestines got punctured, so the surgeons had to reopen my abdomen. They detected some microscopic cancer cells, and I started yet another round of chemo—six months of Doxil and Gemzar this time.

This past summer, eight months after I'd finished the chemo, they found a tumor in my liver. In August I had a part of my liver resected, and I'm still recuperating. I'll be starting six rounds of chemo next week. Once you have ovarian cancer, it's a never-ending cycle of remissions and recurrences.

How do I cope? I have a lot of faith, and I get strength from prayer and from my family's support. And I never think about my illness. Even when I'm having chemo, people tell me, "You don't look sick." I always believe that I'm going to beat this disease.

Because of my experiences, I decided to become a volunteer at SHARE: Self-Help for Women with Breast or Ovarian Cancer (www.sharecancersupport.org). I offer counseling in English or Spanish over the SHARE hotline, because I want to help women who have ovarian cancer not to feel so alone.

I was always shy, but after SHARE sent me to a public speaking class, I went to Philadelphia and spoke before 200 physician assistants. *The Today Show* has taped me speaking to students at Mt. Sinai Medical Center, and I've gone to Washington, DC, to talk with New York Senators Clinton and Schumer about research funding. I also speak to Latina women in Spanish Harlem and Queens.

Every year I visit several medical schools. "Every woman can have these symptoms, but persistent symptoms are a red flag," I tell students. "If a woman has them for more than three weeks, I want you to think about ovarian cancer."

Unfortunately, my story is not unique. I try to live each day of my life as fully as possible. And I am committed to helping other women who face symptoms like mine: I share my personal experiences so that they won't have to go through what I did.

About the author: Carmen Diaz is a mother of two and grandmother of four. For many years she worked at NYU Law School as an administrator before retiring in 2004 after being diagnosed with ovarian cancer. She now volunteers for the Ovarian Cancer National Alliance (www.ovariancancer.org) and the SHARE hotline (866-53SHARE)

Intern's Journal—Convince Me

Jennifer Reckrey
10/17/2008

How do you convince someone to do something they don't really care about?

This week I took care of a fifty-eight-year-old woman who came to the hospital with one week of fevers, diarrhea, burning with urination, and abdominal pain. Though she probably had an infection, the CT scan she got in the ER didn't reveal its source. It did, however, show that something was wrong with her uterus and ovaries. If the odd-looking mass was an abscess, it needed to be drained. If it was a cancer, she needed a very different sort of treatment plan. And to find out what was going on, she needed an MRI.

When I first asked her about it, she quickly agreed. She'd had MRIs scheduled in the past (her outpatient gynecologist was concerned about her too), but had always missed her appointments. She seemed glad for the chance to get this cumbersome test over with while she was stuck in the hospital anyway. But when they called her down for the scan, she refused to go.

I went to her room, where she was resting comfortably on her bed and watching TV. I explained what the test would be like and why it was so important that she get it done as soon as possible. I tried to be gentle yet firm. And she wouldn't budge. When I asked her why she wouldn't go, she said that she didn't want to miss her soap opera. Without knowing how I got there, I found myself playing the bad cop.

"Do you really think watching your telenovela is more important than trying to find where your infection is coming from and making sure that you don't have cancer?" I asked.

"Yes," she answered.

About an hour later, my supervising physician went to talk with her, and she told him that she was afraid of feeling claustrophobic in the MRI machine. Thinking the problem solved, I gave her some encouragement and a sedative to help her relax and sent her for the test. An aide wheeled her down to the radiology suite, but just ten minutes later wheeled her right back up to the floor again. From down the hall, I could hear her complaining that the line for the MRI machine was too long and that she didn't want to wait for yet another test. I left the hospital that day wondering what I could have done differently, better.

When I came in the next morning, she'd had the MRI overnight. No fanfare. No sedation. No big deal. (And no big help either. The MRI confirmed neither abscess nor cancer, and gave no further clue as to what might be causing her pain and fevers.)

There have been many other patients like her this week: the diabetic with the huge, gaping sore on his foot who refused antibiotics and insulin; the young sickle-cell patient who wouldn't go home until her pain cleared completely; the family who insisted that their demented, dying mother have a feeding tube inserted; the chronic schizophrenic, now stable, who refused to take his antipsychotics.

I must respect each individual's right to make decisions about his or her care, but I must also make sure that these patients understand the consequences of the decisions made. My training gives me a perspective on the big picture that patients often don't have. For me to pretend that all options are equally good would be just as dishonest as pretending that, since I'm the doctor, I should have the final say.

Balancing these competing demands—the patient's right to freedom, the doctor's duty to provide guidance—is not easy.

About the author: Jennifer Reckrey MD is a family medicine resident in New York City. Each week while she was an intern, she wrote about her experiences as a brand-new doctor. This story is from week six. "I started writing these reflections to keep in touch with friends and family. But the process of putting my experiences into words has helped me to better understand and develop my own practice of medicine."

in the taxi to the MRI

Rachel Hadas
10/24/2008

I try to concentrate on the weather. Everything
deliquesces into simile.
Sleet ticks onto the windshield like a clock.
Truth blinks on/off like a stuck traffic signal.
It is better to live in the light but the light is flickering.
Anything more than the truth would have seemed too weak-
Poetic paradox understood too late
or maybe just in time. What time is it?
A small white poodle in a quilted coat
lifts a leg to pee against a hydrant
on Sixtieth Street, and we are nearly there,
early, of course. And since (she said) my heart
has been wrung out, no, broken, this is the . . .
this has to be . . . The sentence will not end.
The mind pulls, stretches, struggles, and returns
not to any absolute beginning
but a blank wall. Is there a door in it?
A future? How to get there? And once there
how to escape? When flickering stops and steady
light shines, that may be the worst of all.
Anything more than the truth would have seemed too weak,
but mercifully the blinking begins again.

---

*About the poet: Rachel Hadas is board of governors professor of English, Newark campus,
Rutgers University. The latest of her many books of poems is* The River of Forgetfulness
(David Robert, 2006); Classics *(WordTech Communications), a volume of selected prose,
was published in 2007. Her Web site is www.rachelhadas.com.*

*About the poem: "My husband's MRI signaled the early stages of the process of diagnosing
a progressive dementia. Even before he took the test, I instinctively knew the news would
not be good. Poetry helps me to understand what I am feeling and thinking; it helps me
to not feel overwhelmed and purely reactive. I would be delighted were the poem to prove
of help to anyone."*

Halloween Horrors

Paul Gross
10/31/2008

One October evening last year, I went to our local pharmacy to pick up a prescription for my daughter. I made sure to bring Cara's insurance card because my employer had switched us to a new health plan.

I wasn't sorry about the change. Our prior plan had been operated by incompetents—although they might only have been crooks, I couldn't be sure—who also managed our flexible spending accounts. These accounts, you may recall, collect pre-tax income from your pay and then return it to you to pay for out-of-pocket medical expenses.

With that plan, nothing ever worked as advertised. I would submit a dental bill for reimbursement and the company would review it for three months before sending me a denial notice, stating that my health plan had no dental coverage.

"I know that I have no dental coverage," I'd tell the representative on the phone. "That's why I put a big X in the box labeled Flexible Spending Account."

"You sure did!" she'd say cheerfully. "I don't know why they did that. You'll have to submit it again. This time, put my name on it . . .."

Or I'd submit a claim for a medical expense that was covered, then hear nothing for months and months.

"We've fallen behind," a weary-sounding representative would lament. I could picture the ceiling-high stacks of claim forms swaying on her desk. "You should be hearing shortly . . .."

No one ever said "I'm sorry." No one ever acknowledged the annoyance of the paperwork or the aggravation of waiting on hold for a representative. No one ever said, "Gee whiz! We hoped you wouldn't notice, because if you forget to contact us, we get to keep your money," although I suspected that this was one of their operating strategies.

So I was happy with the change in health plans. And there at the pharmacy, I optimistically produced my daughter's new plastic card.

The pharmacist punched something into a computer and stared impassively at a screen. After several minutes, I wandered off to look at vitamin capsules and cold remedies.

When I returned ten minutes later, the pharmacist was on the phone with my insurance company. Ten minutes after that, he was on hold for a different company, the one that manages the pharmacy plan.

While the pharmacist waited, I browsed the magazine rack. Then I made my way to the Halloween aisle, where I saw candy similar to the trick-or-treat leftovers desiccating in our freezer since the previous October.

The pharmacist finally beckoned and rendered a verdict: "Your daughter isn't covered under your pharmacy plan."

"What?"

"They've got *you* on their system, but no one else in your family."

"I can't believe . . ."

"They say you've got to talk to your benefits representative."

I thanked him for his thirty minutes of trouble. The next day I called my benefits representative, who reassured me that our entire family was in their system. Days later, my wife tried to fill a prescription—no luck.

The following pattern repeated itself over the next few weeks: (1) I'd call my benefits representative and receive assurances that the problem had been fixed; (2) we'd try to fill a prescription for my wife or daughter; and (3) the pharmacist would tell us that she wasn't in the system. Finally, weeks later, somebody somewhere flicked a switch and—*voilà*—the pharmacy plan kicked into place.

Which brings me to the upcoming presidential election.

One of the candidates for our highest office is advocating new deregulations that would encourage Americans to comparison shop for health plans in all fifty states. This is nifty, if your idea of a simpler, more efficient health system is more health plans.

My first reaction was: who has time to spend evenings and weekends comparison shopping for health plans in all fifty states? And who wants to repeat the shopping trip in a year, when a plan's sticker price is sure to go up? Each change in plans, of course, means new cards, new forms, a new list of covered doctors . . ..

The last medical comparison shopping I did was to hunt online for a Medicare Part D prescription drug plan for my 83-year-old mother. It was a nuisance. Years later, she's still using the same plan. Not because it's still the best for her—who knows?—but because it's just simpler that way.

The suggestion that some nimble shopping in a health-plan emporium is going to fix our health-care system would never occur to anyone who's wrangled with prior authorizations, changing doctors when one plan flips to another, or getting inappropriate bills because last year's insurance company was incorrectly charged for this year's blood tests.

Most people understand that each new plan—even a better plan—is a new bureaucracy. One more snarl in a tangled health-care web that already boasts hundreds of commercial health carriers and thousands upon thousands of different plans.

The only person I can imagine embracing a "more-plans-the-merrier" system, aside from insurance investors, is someone to whom it won't apply. Someone like our current presidential candidates—who as senators have a government-financed insurance menu that appears to suit them just fine.

For this Halloween season, the notion that we should flood the nation with more health plans seems like a horror-film plot rather than a long-term strategy for better health care.

Once Halloween is over and we put away the costumes and candy, I could go for fewer health plans. Fewer phone numbers. Less rigmarole. And an end to evenings spent wandering the pharmacy aisles, waiting for an okay from Health Plan Number 3,011.

―――――――――――

About the author: *Paul Gross is editor-in-chief of* Pulse—voices from the heart of medicine.

My patient, my friend

Larry Zaroff
11/7/2008

Death is not always the same. Quantity, fixed: one per patient. Quality, variable.

Doctors see many deaths, of different kinds. This is true of any doctor, whether or not he or she is a surgeon, as I am.

It's easier for the doctor when death is expected, following a long illness, a chronic disease. Harder when it's unforeseen—the heart attack, the accident, the gun shot, the sudden death in a young man or woman who seemed a conqueror.

Sometimes, in a long-term patient-doctor relationship, the two types of death merge: Death becomes the harsh, abrupt end to a journey taken by two travelers.

M was a special patient—thirty-something, warm, charming, brave. At our first meeting, an office visit in the early Sixties, she gave me her special homemade pickles, just to my liking, medium sour with a dill flavor. Over the next decade, she and her family and I became close. She was generous, always patient. The operations I performed to treat her mitral valve disease, a manifestation of previous rheumatic fever, reflected cardiac surgery's progress over that time.

In her first operation, I incised her chest between the ribs on the left side. I opened her calcified blocked mitral valve—the gateway to the left ventricle, which pumps blood to the body—by blindly inserting my finger through the left atrium, the heart's upper chamber, breaking open the valve's fused leaflets.

M was better for five years. I followed her closely at regular intervals until her increasing shortness of breath and fatigue signaled that the valve blockage had recurred. When her cardiologist and I suggested another operation, more complicated than the first, she did not hesitate. And when I explained the greater risk, she smiled and passed the pickle jar across the desk. Her trust, her belief was complete.

I replaced M's diseased valve with a mechanical prosthesis of metal and plastic, this operation done through an incision in the midline dividing the breastbone. She again recovered swiftly, resuming her busy life as a wife and mother.

Another five years of follow-up, of friendship, during which M and I became even closer. We talked about more than just her medical care, kept up with what was happening with each other's families and children.

Ten years after her first heart operation, five years after her second, M came to the office thin and weak, having suffered—and only partially recovered from—two small strokes. Despite her being on blood thinners, small clots were breaking off from the plastic and metal valve and traveling to her brain. She was more frightened than she had ever been, and seriously ill, so sick that she brought no pickles.

Serious consultations followed between patient, family, cardiologist and the surgical team. Reoperations carry greater risks because of the adhesions that join the heart, pericardium (the sac encasing the heart) and surrounding lungs in a mass of scar tissue. An operation to remove M's mechanical prosthesis and replace it with a bioprosthesis—a pig valve, less prone to form clots—posed greater dangers than the first two. She, courageous, had expectations of full recovery.

As Susan Sontag has argued, caring for the very sick has consequences for the physician. Those consequences are magnified when patient and doctor are friends and enjoy a long relationship. I shared M's suffering, her pain; I wanted to help.

The third surgery, through the right chest, was difficult. Extensive adhesions, plus the need to remove the previous valve embedded in the heart muscle, made for an epic procedure.

An epic procedure. And a technical error.

In excising the first prosthesis, I damaged the heart wall. Though I repaired the tear, I feared complications. M was taken to the intensive care unit in stable condition, but a few hours later a massive, sudden bleeding occurred.

My friend M died in the intensive care unit.

Any death in which a doctor participates has a powerful impact. Somehow, when the death is surgical and acute—a hands-on death resulting from a technical error—the onus and the guilt feel greater. Atul Gawande, MD, in his superb book

Complications: A Surgeon's Notes on an Imperfect Science, reminds us that the best doctors in the best hospitals make mistakes, serious blunders that kill people.

I find no solace in knowing this.

Would I have felt less devastated, less depressed, better able to move on to the next patient if M and I had not been friends for ten years? I think yes.

But I would have missed the best part of medical practice—a long relationship, the sharing of an illness, the traveling of a road together.

That is my consolation.

About the author: *Following his residency and two years in the U.S. Army Surgical Research Unit, Larry Zaroff MD PhD has pursued five careers. He focused for twenty-nine years on cardiac surgery, including a stint as director of the cardiac surgical research laboratory at Harvard. There his work centered on the development of the demand pacemaker. He spent the next ten years concentrating on climbing and did a first ascent of Chulu West, a 22,000-foot peak on the Nepal-Tibet border. His third life has been at Stanford University, where he received a PhD in 2000 and where he teaches courses in medical humanities. His fourth career has been as a writer for the* New York Times *science section. He now works one day a week as a volunteer family doctor. He has received awards as the outstanding faculty advisor for the Human Biology program and in 2006 was honored as Stanford's Teacher of the Year.*

little black boy

Jimmy Moss
11/14/2008

little black boy
                              sit down.
fold your hands into your lap
and put your lap into order
now cry me a little song.
sing me a little note about me
caring about what you care about,
then dream me a little dream.
and when your tears turn into
oases and exposed rivers
                              stand up
and pour me a little cup
fill it with every broken promise
and the unfulfilled moments of
belated birthdays and first days
of the school year when your
clothes were unkempt . . . then
tell me a little secret
about how—you wish your father
bothered enough to be a father
or fathered another version of you,
so that you could have a friend
                              and then
write me a little poem.
make me a little rhyme about
the places you lived and the schools
you've attended
the teachers you've impressed
and the classmates
you've offended . . . by simply
being a   little black boy
who could read and speak well
and vividly express himself,
find clean shirts amongst the dirty ones
and dress himself
                              long enough

                              to cover up his little pain
and then bring me a little more
of whatever it is that you have
bundled up in your little hand,
stashed away from piercing eyes,
tucked inside of your little lap
that you peek at every moment
you are given a little slack
a little chance   and little hope
a little grade for your little work
just . . . put it in my hand . . .
and trust me,
                              little black boy
i promise to give it back—in order.

About the poet: *Jimmy Moss is a fourth-year medical student at Florida State University College of Medicine. "I got interested in writing as a way of trying to communicate many of the ineffable aspects of my life. I enjoy writing about various issues (love, poverty, nature, social interactions, etc.) and am always challenging myself to push my creativity to new levels of expansion and understanding."*

About the poem: *"This poem is about me, my upbringing and how awkward I used to feel for wanting (desiring) something more than the options my environment was daily presenting to me. Growing up in poverty wasn't all that hard, because everyone around me was poor. The more difficult tasks were trying to overcome the negative connotations associated with 'being from the 'hood,' acquiring academic enhancement from sub-par school systems, and looking past all of the negativity I received from others for attempting to establish a better existence for myself. I cared about progress and was ridiculed for it.*

"In the poem I mention 'finding clean shirts amongst the dirty ones,' which symbolizes the innocence of how I viewed things—because to me that was more of a skill than get-ting good grades. I had to learn (mostly on my own) that simply surviving wasn't the only thing life was about. I had to visualize myself in a better situation—one where I was exceeding expectations and expanding on numerous levels. However, since I had no blueprint to follow, I had to trust that life was going to take care of my little portion of

hope. I had to have faith that if I at least attempted to do the right things, something or someone (e.g., the narrator of the poem) would meet me halfway, thereby confirming that my dreams, thoughts, hard work, embarrassments, trying times, sacrifices and tears were not in vain.

"So often, I think that individuals who rise above statistical and societal stereotypes are not given enough social support, so they are forced to trust that life itself will not let them down. So far, doing just that has worked out well for me."

HOSPICE

Joanne Wilkinson
11/21/2008

My patient's beagle is very quiet. He lies next to the brown leather living-room chair she used to sit in when I would come to see her at home. His nose is down on his paws, and his round eyes look up at me, up at the nurses, the home health aides, the family members who go back and forth between here and the back bedroom. He is very alert, but silent. He stays perfectly still.

My patient's sons want to know things. How much longer will it be, will she be in pain, what will the end be like, will she be conscious? Should they take the rest of the week off from work, should they call the son in California and ask him to come? Yes, I tell them. Bring the relatives from far away, call in sick to work, get the minister, the undertaker, the cousin with the good voice who wants to sing at the service. It won't be long.

They pace back and forth in the kitchen, stirring the air with their movement. Their footsteps shake the house's foundations. Would it have been different, they ask, if we'd caught it earlier, if she'd had the colonoscopy at fifty like you're supposed to, if she hadn't gone to Europe for two years and not seen a doctor? If they had visited more often, or nagged her about her health, or been nicer to her back in second grade when she told them to finish their homework? No, I tell them, no. Of course not, no.

She first showed up in my office not six months ago, a retired college professor proud of her good health, for a routine physical. Instead of just the cholesterol and HDL, I ordered some other things too—she hadn't seen a doctor in years, and I think of them as the "just in case" labs. A complete blood count. Electrolytes. Just in case she had something bad that no one knew about. And she did—severe anemia, with a hemoglobin of 8.5 when normal is above 12.

We had literally two office visits after that—the one to plan her colonoscopy and the one where we went over her abdominal CT scan studded with metastases—and then I started seeing her at home.

My patient's nurses want to talk strategy with me. This much narcotic, for this long, and the drops that dissolve in the mouth? This many nurses, for this many days, and the oxygen with the bubbles in it so she won't feel too dry? Fine, I tell them, it's all fine, you guys do good work, just show me where to sign and who to call. I trust you.

My patient is quiet, sedated. She appears to be sleeping. I hold her hand when I go in to see her, and I don't use my stethoscope. The humidified oxygen hisses and bubbles gently, sounding like rain. I think of the four home visits we have had—first sitting in the living room looking at family photos together, later sitting on the foot of this bed, talking about getting the oxygen ordered. I've known her such a short time, but like her so much. She does not open her eyes, and I try to imagine what she is dreaming about. Long walks in Paris during her sabbatical year? Playing the piano for Christmas carols with the family? Touching the silky head of her dog? You did good, I tell her quietly. It's okay. You rest now.

In the kitchen, before I leave, I tell them all that I am sorry. That I am only a phone call away, that they can call me at any time and ask to be put straight through. I know, though, that they won't, that my work here is done. In another hour I'll be back in my office prescribing birth-control pills for college students and cleaning wax out of ears and diagnosing allergic rhinitis—and remembering the watchful silence in that house, the tick of the kitchen clock under the fluorescent lights, the silky ears of the beagle as he mourns.

About the author: Joanne Wilkinson MD MSc decided to be a doctor when she was eight so that she could support her writing habit. "I told my pediatrician that I was going to be a writer, but that in order to make money I would be a doctor 'during the day.' He laughed ... now I know why." Since then, Joanne has attended and led multiple writing workshops and has had short stories and essays published. Along the way, she graduated from medical school and practiced full-time for six years; she is now a member of the academic/research faculty at Boston University Medical School.

Thanksgiving Reflections

Pulse *Writers and Editors*
11/28/08

Editor's note: This Thanksgiving tugs hard at the emotions. While an economic gale roils the world, our freshly chosen captain stands on deck, pointing out a new direction for our battered ship of state. At the same time, each of us has personal joys and sorrows to contemplate. We asked Pulse's *writers and editors to take a moment to share their reflections.*

This year, I am thankful for my four quirky little grandsons, my three loving children and my beloved husband of almost forty years. I am especially thankful that the country we share has a chance to find its way again and to call all of us, young and old, toward a future that can still be bright and full of promise. —*Johanna Shapiro*

I'm thankful for my daughter, and for how she kicks and growls in delight when I enter her room at 6 a.m. —*Joanne Wilkinson*

As one who came of political age in the 1960s, I remember as only a young man can the losses of JFK, RFK and MLK. As an older man, I'm all too aware of the fragility of any single human life. But I will be grateful this Thanksgiving for the resurrection of hope, and of a revolutionary spirit I haven't experienced in over forty years. —*Rick Flinders*

In my sixties, after a decade marked by loss (my husband, my sister, both parents, several friends) and change (home, job, rhythm of life), I find myself waking up and going to sleep with the words "Thank you" as my only prayer. I don't know where this gratitude comes from, what it's for or to whom or what it's directed. I only know that it's my response to this life and carries me through each day with a keen sense of wonder. —*Veneta Masson*

I decided to ask my 13-year-old son Sean, who has autism, what he is thankful for. He made a list:

1. I'm thankful that my birthday is before my dad's.
2. I'm thankful that my shoe size is now 10½ and dad's is only 9.
3. I'm thankful that my hand is bigger than daddy's.
4. I'm thankful that I can beat my daddy at arm wrestling (I let him win sometimes).
5. I'm thankful that I can play the drums and the trumpet and my dad can't.
6. I'm thankful that I can swim faster than my dad.

7. I'm thankful that my mom and dad will make a turkey for me on Thanksgiving.

(Thanks, Sean! I hope there aren't too many growth spurts left. :-)

—*John Harrington*

This past week, one of our first-year medical students died—a suicide. We're all in shock, and the students, in particular, are devastated. This event took me to a lot of sad places, including the time that I was severely depressed and nearly ended my life. Today I am grateful for those who were there when I needed them and helped me put my life back together: my wife Marsha, Dr. Jim Zettel and, in their own inimitable way, my children Annie and Tom. —*Warren Holleman*

A haiku:
our life on the bay—
waves washed with sun, rain, or fog,
grateful for it all.

—*Neal Whitman and Elaine Weiss*

I'm most thankful this year that we elected a man who is intelligent and articulate, believes in social justice and appears to reject preemptive war and torture. Yes, change has come to America, thank God. —*Barry Thompson*

I am so thankful for my two kids (Alice, 11, and Jimmie, 8) and for their understanding and gentleness. Alice and Jimmie often offer to give me a massage when my back hurts at the end of the day. For me, hearing "Mommy, is this the right spot?" or "How about this spot, Mommy?" is better than any medication. —*Jan Qiu*

I am thankful that my family and I have our health and are happy in our pursuits, and that I still love practicing medicine. We are also thankful that we have a new president who demonstrates competence and vision and offers us hope for the future. —*Sandy Brown*

I am thankful for the good brain chemistry that enables me to get through pain and suffering by listening to my favorite music. This year, I am especially thankful to the American people for electing Barack Obama and to the Pulitzer Prize people for giving Bob Dylan a special award! —*Beth Hadas*

I would simply like to offer a prayer and thanks for all things dear and familiar, which was my personal prayer on 9/11/01. —*Ann Weiss*

Here are people and things I'm thankful for:
My maternal grandmother for her advice about parenting: "Do the best you can, and hope they don't end up in prison."
My paternal grandmother for her advice about wealth: "It's not very far from corn pone to plum pudding, but it's a long way back."
My mother for her advice about love: "Don't be kissing at the gate. Love may be blind, but the neighbors ain't."
And my son (then age 8) for his advice about fatherhood: "You're a lot nicer since you quit delivering babies." —*John Scott*

I am especially thankful to *Pulse* for making a home for stories and poems in and about medicine. —*Howard Stein*

My mother taught me so much, so early and so unknowingly (on my part). The teaching was like a lovely redbird in flight. I often stop and wonder, "Where did that come from?" My flights of fancy and creativity and my grounding in solid values go right back to that dear source, my mother. I was blessed.

Early Bird Preparation

This morning from the kitchen window
I watch the redbird come and go.
Though night hangs dark on my shoulders,
I recall my mother saying it was
                    good luck, seeing a redbird.
I believed her then and believe her now.

When I kneel to pray, to say thank you,
I think of her and luck. Grateful to her.

I have had big agendas and laptop plans,
Drunk champagne flying first class, spitting
out marketing templates with ease, photos of
husband, daughter, grandsons in a briefcase.
                              Oh! I was flying then!
But when I kneel to pray, to say thank you,
I am grateful to her for seeing what is real.
Grateful to her for luck and good preparation.

—*Judy Schaefer*

Running out of Metaphors

Howard F. Stein
12/5/2008

His rapidly metastasizing cancer
was not his only problem:
He was not only running out
of life, he was running out of metaphors.
Metaphors had sustained him
for the four months since
they discovered the spot.
He started out
losing weight as "The Incredible
Shrinking Man"; then he became
Gregor Samsa for a while;
briefly he was the consumptive Violetta,
soon followed by Ivan Ilych.
He even remembered Susan Sontag
and Solzhenitsyn and so railed
at his wasting. He leaped
from metaphor to metaphor the way
a stone skips over water. He asked
all the questions everyone asks,
but felt no comfort from
the answers.
Companions and kin beset him
like Job's friends. He graciously refused
their unctuous offerings, their leaden words.
Thinking could no longer save him.
His only balm now was his love for his son.
He had at last found something that had no metaphor:
This time, love would have to be enough.

About the poet: *Howard Stein PhD, a psychoanalytic and medical anthropologist, is a professor in the Department of Family and Preventive Medicine at the University of Oklahoma Health Sciences Center in Oklahoma City, where he has taught for thirty years. A poet as well as a researcher and scholar, he has published five books of poetry, including* Theme and Variations *(Finishing Line Press, 2008). In 2006 he was nominated for Oklahoma Poet Laureate.*

About the poem: *"As patients, family members and health care professionals, we are constantly 'making sense' out of disease and illness. These meanings often take the form of metaphors, one of many figures of speech that speak of likeness, resemblance and identity. Long a teacher of physician-patient relationships, I 'imagined' myself into one of our cases and through writing the poem came to realize that through metaphor we can bring life and death near—or push them away. Metaphor can shut out as well as let in. When my poetic protagonist had exhausted his literary imagination, what remained was his deep love for his son, a relationship he would soon lose in dying."*

A view from Nepal

Caroline Jones
12/12/2008

The farmer wanted to know why his three-year-old son couldn't walk or talk.

I sat opposite him in a dark, cold classroom converted into an examination room for a four-day medical clinic last spring in the village of Lapa, high in the Himalayas.

Wind whistled through the stone walls; rain pounded on the tin roof. The room's single ceiling bulb kept flickering and dying; I had to use a camping headlamp to see my notes. And communications were hampered, to say the least: We conversed via two translators—from English to Nepali, from Nepali to the local Tamang language, then back again. It sounded a bit like the telephone game, and had similarly uncertain results.

Still, one look was all I needed to make the diagnosis: Down syndrome. I found the telltale single hand crease, eye folds and wide gap between the first and second toes and asked about the boy's medical history: he'd never seen a doctor; sometimes he had diarrhea, fever or a cough.

I thought back to my journey here, the last leg of which had begun five days earlier. With two other doctors, I had left Nepal's capital, Kathmandu, on a winding, bumpy, eight-hour Jeep ride up into the Ganesh Himal range. As we drove higher, the sheer mountainside drops grew more terrifying, but we didn't notice them much, mesmerized as we were by the stunning views and the farmhouses hanging off the nearly vertical terraced hillsides. At day's end, we joined the field team who would take us the rest of the way to Lapa—a four-day trek by foot.

Our trip had been organized by Himalayan HealthCare, an independent, nonsectarian nonprofit cofounded by Anil Parajuli, a Nepalese trek operator.

Nepal, sandwiched between Tibet and India, is one of the world's poorest countries. Since its royal family was wiped out by a murder-suicide in 2001, it's been torn by clashes between an unpopular monarchy and insurgent Maoists, with killings, disappearances and detentions on both sides. The majority of Nepal's people are subsistence farmers living in inhospitable mountain villages like Lapa. Himalayan HealthCare aids several such villages, using its shoestring budget to fund medical treks, train villagers as health-care workers and teachers, provide for orphans and foster commercial projects such as handicrafts and cardamom-growing.

Each day of our trek to Lapa, we hiked steep, switchback trails up to 14,000-foot-high mountain passes, only to descend the other side and camp overnight in the valley below. The next morning, we'd ascend again. Our staff, cooks and porters greatly eased the journey by carrying our gear and making us comfortable in our tents, delivering sweet chai tea first thing in the morning and a hot water bottle at night.

As we carried our day packs, the diminutive Nepalese porters went on ahead lugging our dining table and chairs, stove and kerosene supplies. They bent double under their *dokas*, overloaded bamboo baskets supported by bands across their foreheads. Many wore only flip-flops; a few, wearing no shoes at all, left naked footprints in the snow.

Lapa badly needed health care, having had none in the four years since its sole health-care worker was kidnapped by Maoists and held prisoner with a string of grenades around his neck. (After Himalayan HealthCare paid his $300 ransom, he left.) Many of our patients had never left their villages or been examined by a doctor. Their most common complaints—painful knees and breathlessness while climbing—were the legacy of lifetimes spent carrying heavy burdens long distances and dwelling in wood-smoke-filled houses.

We saw a wide range of ailments, from tuberculosis of the lymph nodes to chronic ear infections, gastritis, worm infestations, severe cataracts, stroke, rheumatoid arthritis and asthma or chronic obstructive lung disease. But in most cases, the only treatment we could offer was enough acetaminophen or ibuprofen to provide a few weeks of relief. We sent a few serious cases to the hospital in Dhading besi, three days away, but only if the patient could make the trip on foot—or carried in a *doka* (our "basket cases").

I looked at the man in front of me. He was a typical Nepalese farmer—tiny in stature, weather-beaten, shy, gentle, patient, worn down by life. "Down syndrome" . . . "genetic abnormality" . . . "chromosomes" . . . these words would hold no meaning for him. Mainly, I reasoned, he just needed to know whether there was something horribly wrong with his son. It was unlikely that the boy would ever go to school, but he would grow up to farm alongside his parents. I reassured the man that his son eventually would walk and talk, and gave the boy a multivitamin and an empiric treatment for intestinal worms.

We parted with small smiles, a slight mutual bow and a simple "Namaste," pressing our own palms together as if in prayer. I wondered what the man thought of our encounter; I hoped that he came away feeling more hopeful.

In all, my colleagues and I saw 450 people in Lapa, working far into the final evening. It was difficult to feel that we'd given them much. But perhaps our offers of Band-Aid medicine and modest comfort meant more than we realized. Our patients' "Namaste" always sounded thankful, and they did seem grateful to be seen and listened to.

We in turn had been challenged physically and mentally, walked the Himalayan foothills and had the privilege of sharing the lives of the Tamang people. An outsider in a community so different from my own, I felt welcomed and accepted by my patients in a deeply personal way. As they confided their intimate concerns to me, I felt strongly connected to them. And in this remote setting, far from the daily hassles of American health care, I felt my love of medicine renewed.

This was their gift to me.

About the author: Caroline Jones MD is a family physician on the faculty at Saint Joseph's Medical Center Family Medicine Residency Program in Yonkers, NY. She has participated in medical missions to Ghana and Nepal. "I have always found that traveling to a different part of the world to work in that culture is a rewarding experience. Medicine is amazing in that it allows me to step into other people's worlds, to ask them important questions about their lives and to appreciate their strengths and their struggles."

Ripped from the Headlights

Maureen Picard Robins
12/19/2008

"Get a notebook," he said.

Dr. Altman and I stood face to face on the pediatric surgical floor of Columbia-Presbyterian Babies & Children's Hospital. It was the first week in December. A metal crib—it seemed more like a cage or prison—separated us. In this center space lay my yellow heart: my eight-week-old daughter, wounded by surgery, dulled by morphine, our whispers flying over her.

It had been nearly twenty-four hours since Dr. Altman opened the baby's abdomen and held her tiny intestines in his hands, untwisting them like a fisherman untangling his line; nearly one day since he'd performed a Kasai procedure, fashioning a conduit so that bile could tremble down to her small intestine; one thousand four hundred and forty minutes since I'd been ripped from the headlights of the speeding car known as biliary atresia, a rare condition in which the duct from the liver to the small intestine is blocked or missing.

"There's a lot to learn," Dr. Altman said. "Write down all your questions. There is no way you will remember all this."

There was only one question I wanted to ask, and I didn't dare.

Besides that, there were so many other things I didn't know. I didn't know how long it would take for her jaundice to clear, or if it ever would. I didn't know what to do if it didn't clear. I didn't know what cholangitis is. (It's an infection in the bile duct, I learned; but I also didn't know if I'd recognize an infection.) I didn't know if her liver would regenerate from its "insult." I didn't know if I could trust my pediatrician anymore. Or myself.

Dr. Altman told me that about a third of babies who have Kasai procedures do well, period. About a third only partially clear their jaundice and eventually need a liver transplant. Another third don't make it at all.

I got a notebook.

I wrote everything down.

Seven days later, the baby was well enough to leave the hospital, although we wouldn't know the outcome of her Kasai for at least a month. In the meantime, Dr. Altman arranged for me to take her to see a pediatric gastroenterologist, Dr. Joseph Levy. I wrote down all my questions.

"Will Jackie live?" I wrote.

The next day, shivering in Dr. Levy's office, I undressed the baby, who promptly peed neon-green liquid into the cup of my hand. "It's all right," Dr. Levy said, meaning not to worry about the floor—but at that moment he knew that she would fall into one of the unlucky thirds, and he knew that I knew.

Dr. Levy asked to see my notebook questions. He answered them as best he could and wrote down instructions: how to trick a baby into eating bitter powdered medicine; how to feed her sweet potatoes on a nipple; how to dispense fat-soluble vitamins and a prophylactic antibiotic. He told me that he would phone me every night between 8:00 and 10:00 to see how we were doing, and that I should bring the baby back in two days. The next two weeks were critical, he said, and Jackie was fragile.

I got smarter. Through Dr. Levy and others, I met mothers of children who'd had biliary atresia and liver transplants. Until then, I had only read about liver transplants in newspaper headlines. Now I researched and cried my way through medical textbooks and journals while my husband, Wayne, took care of my older daughter, Elizabeth, and the household. The hue of Jackie's skin, urine and excretions told me that her first surgery was only a partial success, buying time. "The numbers are not going down," I wailed to Dr. Levy on the phone one night. "She's still yellow!"

A month post-Kasai, I took the baby back to Dr. Altman.

He counseled me to decide on a path and put all my trust in it. If something went wrong, I needed to be in a place where I could say, "I tried my best." No second guessing. No regrets. At that moment, I couldn't comprehend the picture he was painting. I couldn't even comprehend my own psyche: one minute I was humming lullabies, the next I was mentally boxing with God. But I agreed to take the baby to yet another specialist, Dr. Stephen Dunn in Philadelphia, to be evaluated for a liver transplant.

We drove to see Dr. Dunn the following week. He placed Jackie on the list, and we started our wait.

Dr. Levy continued to call me every night and to see Jackie weekly, but the struggle to keep her alive only intensified as we waited. She could not sit. She could not eat. And if she did, it came back at me. Her liver, sensing its own failure, grew to compensate. Her tiny belly swelled with liver and fluid. She had a herniated belly button.

Still we waited.

She itched all over. She could no longer hold her head up or gather the strength to roll over. I learned to insert a feeding tube, and Dr. Levy prescribed a powerful nutritional liquid to be pumped into her belly. One day in June, I said goodbye to Dr. Levy before he went on vacation.

That next evening, at the time when he usually called, the phone rang.

It was Dr. Dunn, calling to say, "Come, we have a liver for Jackie."

About the author: Maureen Picard Robins is a poet and writer and an assistant principal in New York City. Her collection of poems Transmigration of Souls *was published this year by Finishing Line Press. She coauthored* The Good Teacher Mentor *(Teachers College Press, 2003). She recently edited an anthology of original essays for a collection,* The Pressures of Teaching *(Kaplan, 2010). Jackie attends high school.*

winter

Tree Years

Addeane Caelleigh
12/26/2008

We used to trade off,
she said.

He hated trees dying in our living room.
I always loved the blue spruces
decorated on my December birthday

But his father fell near theirs
dying in their living room
one childhood night.

So we'd have a year with tangled lights, a crooked stand
      he sometimes helped me put together
Then a year with presents stacked on the corner table,
      with no dry needles to sweep.

Turn and turn again
a solstice pendulum.
A ring for each alternating year

That was before the fog that eats my life,
some years feast, none famine,
always a forecast of more

She says, I think now
he'd welcome any tree, any year.

About the poet: *After many years as editor of the journal* Academic Medicine, *Addeane Caelleigh is now associate editor of* Hospital Drive *(hospitaldrive.med.virginia.edu), an online journal of literature and art published by the University of Virginia School of Medicine, where she is also an administrator and a teacher of faculty development. Addeane is also curator of* Reflections, *an interdisciplinary humanities exhibit series at the university's Claude Moore Health Sciences Library.*

About the poem: "Tree Years *was prompted by thoughts of how chronic disease insinuates itself into our lives, changing relationships, reshaping inner lives and shifting the patterns of everyday living.*"

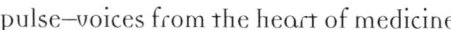

snowscape

Jeffrey R. Steinbauer
1/2/2009

The snowstorm had started on Friday, before I'd gone on call for my group. At first I'd thought the weekend would remain quiet, that the small town where I practiced might just slumber under a fresh blanket of snow. But by early Saturday morning, things had gotten busy at the hospital. Several emergency-room visits, phone calls and admissions from the nursing home changed the stillness I'd felt amid the snowfall. In no time, there was the familiar stress of trying to bring order to a day that was rapidly becoming chaotic.

Sometime that afternoon, I looked up from a chart to see the town sheriff standing at the nursing station. Although we were acquainted through weekly Rotary Club meetings, he now was barely recognizable—bundled in heavy winter clothing, his head covered by a parka hood. Flakes of snow lingered on his jacket and caked his boots. Beneath the hooded parka, his eyes were severe and his face ruddy; together they broadcast an unspoken weather report. He was not smiling.

"Doc, we need you to come with us," he said.

This was an unusual request, coming at an inconvenient time. There was much to be done—phone calls to answer, patients to admit and emergencies to attend to. Thoughts of how to avoid this new, unknown task shot through my mind. But my words came out differently: "What do you need me for?"

"We've found a corpse down by the river. The coroner is out of town, and you're covering for him."

Residency hadn't prepared me for this. The sheriff's earnest voice conveyed that this particular duty was unavoidable. Any chance of getting home to a warm dinner began to melt like the snow on his parka.

Leaving instructions with the nurses, I joined him in the patrol car, leaving behind the lights and bustling noises of the emergency room as we drove to the cold, calm, white outskirts of town. The sky was overcast, the temperature bitterly cold. Snow continued to fall silently, and the countryside gradually took on the appearance of a holiday greeting card. The whole scene, so reminiscent of my pleasant childhood days in the north, jarred against our grim mission.

The sheriff said little, but indicated that they'd found a dead woman near the river. Before she could be taken from the scene, I was legally required, as acting coroner, to investigate and rule on the cause of death.

A few miles out of town, the patrol car turned off the highway and crunched through snowy tracks left by other vehicles. We arrived at a clearing on the river-bank. Stepping from the car, I saw an old Chevrolet pickup truck, the kind favored by local farmers. People stood nearby, looking vaguely familiar in their heavy garb; I recognized the deputy and two people from the local funeral home. Another patrol car and a hearse idled quietly, white fumes rising from their tailpipes.

Feeling out of place and unsure of myself, I walked alone to the truck and opened the door. Inside, behind the wheel, sat a woman perhaps thirty-five years old. She was cold and dead. Her skin had taken on a blue-gray tone that matched the truck interior. The sheriff had said she was the wife of a local farmer known to me only by name. On the floor of the truck cab stood a small charcoal grill, holding some partially burned charcoal.

Although I'd never been trained in forensic medicine, the routine behaviors of a physician took over. I made note of her position, looked for signs of a struggle, noted that the truck windows were rolled up and that the charcoal hadn't burned completely, and proceeded to examine the body. History and physical. I tried to remember from pathology classes the stages of rigor mortis and noted the extent to which it had set in. I didn't undress her, but made a mental note to check her degree of lividity back at the funeral home.

With the truck windows tightly closed, I thought, she'd probably died from asphyxiation as the burning charcoal replaced the cab's oxygen with carbon monoxide. But as I grew more convinced of the cause of death, warm clinical certainty surrendered to cold unknowns. Had she purposely started the charcoal and kept the windows closed to kill herself? Had she come to the river for some quiet time away from a hectic household and mistakenly used the charcoal for warmth?

How had she felt, coming to this place? Had she intended to go home?

I studied her face. It was cold and peaceful in death; there was no anguish, no pain. The cold seeped into my body as it had into hers, my thoughts and feelings now as frozen as the landscape.

After the examination, I released the body to the men from the funeral home, and they put it into the hearse. The landscape looked grayer and the air felt colder as I paused by the riverbank, wondering. Was it suicide or an accident? I would never be sure, but I knew that I would officially call it an accident. As I stood there alone, no holiday greetings came to mind. It was a cold, harsh world where living breath froze in the gentle silence of snowfall.

I felt caught in a world between life and death, caught in the snowscape. She had passed this way a short time before, but she had gone on by a different path. I turned and walked back to the waiting figures. Back to light and warmth. Back to the life of the town.

About the author: Family physician Jeffrey R. Steinbauer MD is a professor at Baylor College of Medicine and medical director of a private practice at the Baylor Clinic. "I come from a family of artists: my father is a professor of music, my son is a documentary film-maker, and my daughter is a creative writer for an educational software company. I've always had artistic interests and worked my way through school as a jazz musician. After I began family practice, those artistic interests shifted to writing about the interesting people and experiences I encountered in medicine. Thinking in terms of the patient's story helps me to see more than guidelines, test values and a problem list when I'm working with patients."

first Night call

Abby Caplin
1/9/2009

During my first night on call as an intern, I felt scared. Not just scared—terrified. I was serving on the medical center's pediatric oncology floor, and medical school hadn't prepared me for children with cancer. What did I know about cutting-edge chemotherapy regimens? What if a child suddenly developed an overwhelming infection or a seizure triggered by a tumor? Someone would expect me to know what to do.

"It's okay," said Brad, the second-year resident. "The nurses do everything. You just treat the kids' hypertension."

"How?" I asked.

"Hydralazine," he answered, glancing at his watch. He looked tired and ready to split. "Ten to twenty milligrams IV every four hours." When I looked up from my hasty scribbling, he was gone. I was alone.

For reassurance, I touched the small but reliable pediatric handbook in my white coat pocket. My other pocket was stuffed with index cards, each labeled with a patient's name, diagnosis and quantities of information written in my tiny print.

I looked down the hall towards the spill of light at the nursing station, the darkening corridors lined with rooms of sick children all trying to sleep—or at least not vomit from the chemotherapy.

I just wanted to go home. I thought about hiding out in the call room and pretending to sleep. I felt nauseated myself. Had I even eaten dinner?

One of the evening nurses emerged from her station. My heart quickened.

"Dr. Caplin," she said firmly, "we have a young patient who's expected to die tonight. You have to speak with the parents. His room is at the end of the hall. His name is Robert."

I found his index card: sixteen years old, three years of leukemia, transferred from somewhere in the Midwest. At checkout, nobody had mentioned anything to me about Robert's dying. How unfair! Wasn't this important enough to tell me? I felt at a loss, inadequate, let down by my supervisors—and by my useless index cards.

"I'm not sure what I'm supposed to do. What do I say to them?" The nurse studied me for a moment. "Just check in and see if they need anything." She hesitated, then added, "You can offer to bring them coffee."

I took a deep breath and headed down the hall. The lights of Houston twinkled through the end window; I wistfully imagined my cozy apartment, then knocked gently at the door and entered.

Robert lay in his hospital bed, peacefully unconscious thanks to the medications dripping through his IV. His mother and father sat in chairs on either side of him. Except for the lights from his heart monitor and the distant city, the room was dark. When his mother turned on the soft background lighting, I saw that Robert was strikingly handsome despite his baldness and pallor, looking more a man than a child. Somehow, from beneath the oxygen mask, IV tubing and monitoring wires, he conveyed a sense of deep inner strength.

I had expected his parents to be distraught. Instead, they seemed remarkably composed. I wondered how they were managing.

"Hello," I began. "I'm Dr. Caplin. I'm so sorry to hear about Robert." They both thanked me for coming. For some reason, they reminded me of the parents of a high-school friend. Suddenly I understood that they were normal people caught in a horrifyingly abnormal situation.

"Can I get you anything? Some coffee?" I asked.

"Oh yes, thank you, Doctor. That would be wonderful, actually," Robert's mother nodded, holding back tears.

Relieved at having something to do, I went to the nurses' station and poured the hospital-issue, slightly burnt coffee into two paper cups. When I returned, both parents jumped out of their chairs and busied themselves with sugar packets and coffee whitener. Seasoned medical parents, they seemed to know that I was a young resident.

They clearly welcomed my presence. They wanted to know where I was from; they wanted to talk. Robert was a terrific son, they said—their youngest, and so capable, with a quick mind and sense of humor. He'd helped them run the family farm.

They said that the pain they felt was unbearable, but they also felt resigned. They wanted Robert's suffering to be over. They planned to fly back to Iowa in the morning; we all knew what they meant by that.

When it came time for me to leave, they shook my hand, and Robert's father said, "We wish you the best of luck in your career, Dr. Caplin. We know you'll make a fine pediatrician." I felt surprised and grateful. Only years later would I fully appreciate the power of his words. I left, encouraging them to have the nurse page me if they needed me.

The nurse, for her part, told me that my work was done, and that she wouldn't disturb me for Robert's expected death.

My beeper went off at 6 a.m. Instead of reviewing the labs and charts of fifteen children, I hurried down the hall to Robert's room.

Sunlight poured in through the windows. The bed was stripped, and his parents were gone. I felt the shock of death's finality; I would never see this family again. In the empty room, not even a coffee cup remained.

What does remain, more than twenty-five years later, is the tremendous gift Robert's parents gave me that night: the knowledge that even in the face of death I could still be of help, and that my willingness to be present as a person could matter as much as any medical intervention. They gave me a deep belief in myself—that I really would become a good doctor. And they conferred it freely, unknowingly and with such grace.

I'll always be grateful, too, to the nurse who took a risk and suggested to a young doctor an unconventional yet potent treatment: the simple offer of a cup of coffee.

About the author: *Abby Caplin MD MA practices mind–body medicine and counseling in San Francisco (www.abbycaplinmd.com; abby@abbycaplinmd.com). Her own personal encounter with autoimmune illness has provided Dr. Caplin, a former pediatrician and allergy–immunology specialist, with a unique opportunity to understand her patients' experiences. Through individual and group counseling, she helps people living with chronic illness and medical conditions to lead empowered and vibrant lives.*

Apologies

Alex Okun
1/16/2009

You were right.
That IV was no good.
Looking at his arm all swollen like that,
I thought, "That says it all."

I'm sorry we kept bothering you.
"Please don't wake him for vitals,"
You told us.

Sometimes we don't see the signs.

I was hoping she would stay home longer,
That you would have had more time together.
She liked starting school every September.
She loved that backpack.

I'm sorry it always took so long
To get into the room.
I'm sorry I took so long to call you back.
I liked our long talks.

If I say "we,"
Then maybe I'm not to blame.
We don't know why some children
Develop this complication.

We don't know why
The brain is so fragile,
Yet so enduring.
That's not very nice.

We don't know why
It happened.
I know you had some ideas.
So did they.

Remember the time
We didn't start the dopamine?
She pulled through that fine,
Amused at our discussions.

Or the time
We got the antibiotics started so fast,
And his blood culture grew out
Only a few hours later?

Those storms down South were nothing
Like what hits you every day.
The levees keep on breaking.
Who can ride these waves of grief?

We remember her.
We will never forget him,
Or you,
Or when we were together.

I just want you to remember
That we still care.

About the poet: Alex Okun MD is associate professor of clinical pediatrics at Albert Einstein College of Medicine and Montefiore Medical Center, and codirector of Pediatric Palliative Care at the Children's Hospital of Montefiore. "I care for kids who are healthy as well as those with special health-care needs, teach residents and students and lead a home visit program for residents. I maintain my own wellness through family closeness and fitness activities."

About the poem: "I wrote and read this poem for our hospital's annual memorial service, 'Always in Our Hearts.' The poem was inspired by the children I've cared for as they were dying, and by their families."

chemo? no, thanks

Elaine Whitman
1/23/2009

"If I were you," said the radiologist, as I sat on the gurney discreetly wiping goo from my right breast, "I'd make an appointment with a breast surgeon as soon as possible." His somber tone of voice, the white blotch radiating ugly spider tendrils on his ultrasound screen . . . neither of these made me nervous. If anything, I felt mild interest: "How very odd. He must think I have breast cancer. Or something."

Ten days later, after a lumpectomy and sentinel lymph node biopsy, my husband and I sat in the breast surgeon's office. "I'm so sorry," he said. "You have Stage IIb breast cancer. There's a 1.1 cm tumor in your right breast, and the cancer has spread to three of your lymph nodes."

I looked first at his solemn face, then around the room. Who was he talking to? I believe the psychological term is "dissociation": a defense mechanism against painful emotions. Oddly, I didn't feel particularly frightened—just very, very tired. Neal drove me home, and I took a five-hour nap.

When I woke up, I realized it was true. I had breast cancer.

Three days later, barely recovered from the lumpectomy, I had a second surgery to remove another cluster of lymph nodes (good news: all clear). "That surgery wasn't so bad," I chirped as I squeezed clear yellow fluid from the drain that dangled below my armpit. "I can handle this."

And then, in the oncologist's office, I heard the dread word "chemo." With no experience of cancer among my family or friends, I knew only one thing about this treatment: it was always discussed in grim whispers. I was suddenly, sickeningly terrified. Neal held me as I sobbed, "I'm not afraid of losing my hair . . . I'm afraid of losing my dignity." I imagined uncontrollable vomiting. Unbearable pain. Writhing in bed as Neal watched, horrified, unable to help me. It was these images, not the fear of dying, that made my heart pound. My terror, I realized, was of losing control. And the only way I could make it through was to take some of that control back.

As a writer, I believe strongly in the power of words. Over the next few days, I thought about chemo. An ugly sound: kee-mow. Being mowed down by a viciously sharp-beaked Kee monster, a cross between a vulture and a velociraptor. "We won't call it chemo," I announced firmly, as much to myself as to Neal. "We'll call it chemo*therapy*, and we'll say it like we mean it. It's medicine. It's going to save my life."

I read everything I could find about chemotherapy. I came across the concept of visualization: picture the chemicals killing the cancer cells, imagine them as little submarines firing torpedoes. Well, fine, but I'm essentially a pacifist. How could I go to war against my own body? Besides, it seemed to me that if I were a cancer cell being attacked by a torpedo, I'd find a quiet spot behind the liver and simply hide until the battle was over. Then I'd come out and multiply like crazy.

So, after some thought, I created a different metaphor. I had always been fond of Cinderella's plump little fairy godmother. At the start of each chemotherapy infusion, I imagined hundreds of miniature fairy godmothers wielding tiny magic wands, floating through my bloodstream searching for cancer cells. Whenever they discovered one they would gaily call out "Bibbidi-bobbidi-boo!" and transform it into . . . a rose. As the other cancer cells realized what was happening, I reasoned, they would come running. After all, who would want to be an—ugh—cancer cell when you could be a beautiful rose? People hate cancer cells. They love roses. Operating on the assumption that everyone (even a cancer cell) wants to be loved, I sent my fairy godmothers to offer the gift of transformation.

It became a group project. Neal bought me a book filled with lush pictures of roses; I flipped through its pages the night before each infusion. I bought myself a gaudy ring adorned with a big honking rose. Friends sent rose paraphernalia: soap, lotion and greeting cards. Everyone learned to say chemo*therapy* . . . and seemed to mean it. After the first infusion, my terror subsided: My oncologist prescribed medications that eliminated nausea and managed pain. I wrapped my Hermès scarves around my bald head and wore blusher every day. My dignity occasionally slipped a bit (as did the scarves), but it never crumbled.

I visualized fairy godmothers. And roses. I never called it chemo. Did any of this make a difference? I have no proof, but I'm convinced that it did. The treatment was hard (four months of biweekly five-hour infusions, an intravenous cocktail of three medications whose side effects included fatigue, diarrhea, mouth sores, muscle aches and bone pain). But it truly wasn't horrible. I believe that choosing my own word, creating my own metaphor, helped. It gave me a critical feeling of control.

I have been in remission for two-and-a-half years. I no longer think about roses or fairy godmothers. I exercise, eat a healthy diet, get regular exams and cherish every day. But, should the time come, I'll take the magic wand out of storage. The metaphor will be waiting for me. And I'll never call it chemo.

About the author: *Elaine Whitman EdD is professor emeritus in the Department of Family and Preventive Medicine at the University of Utah School of Medicine, where she taught students and faculty how to identify and support patients who were experiencing domestic abuse. Her 2005 breast cancer diagnosis put that work in her rearview mirror; she now plays the Native American flute for hospice patients and is a volunteer archivist at Robinson Jeffers Tor House in Carmel, California. She also enjoys bird-watching, hiking, knitting, hand spinning and painting.*

Intern's Journal—surprises

Jennifer Reckrey
1/30/2009

Week Nine

I dreaded my rotation in the Intensive Care Unit. Though all the tools to keep a body alive are right there, their continuous bells and beeps jangle my nerves. I'm always afraid that in this place I will be called on to act decisively and invasively. And my mind will go blank. I will hesitate, and that hesitation will make an already awful situation worse. But even more than that, I dreaded this rotation because I think of the ICU as a dead end—a place you don't leave alive, or if you do, it's as a shadow of your former self.

So when I met my first ICU patient—a sixty-year-old woman with metastatic lung cancer, intubated for respiratory failure after a routine chest-tube placement—I imagined the worst.

She was fully conscious and mentally sharp. For the first two days I cared for her, she was very stable. But she wasn't improving—any time we turned down the ventilator to allow her to take over even a little bit of her own breathing, she struggled for air.

"When will the tube come out?" she wrote on a tablet of paper at her bedside.

I answered honestly: "When, and if, your body is ready."

After having the weekend off, I returned to the ICU to find my patient in bed, still intubated. I imagined that I would spend the afternoon in the often inevitable end-of-life conversation about tracheal tubes and feeding tubes—the conversation that she'd never had with her oncologist. Then, on rounds, the nurse told us that yesterday she had tolerated the lower ventilator settings for almost three hours. We quickly decided that today was the day to try removing the tube. And we did.

What I found most amazing was her voice. A bit hoarse, yes, but strong, with a lilting Island accent. Each sentence ended with a broad smile. She told me that she had always known that this was going to turn out fine. God wasn't ready for her yet; she wasn't ready for him, either.

She also told me not to tell her daughter that the tube was out, because she wanted her daughter, when she walked through the ICU doors, to find her sitting up in bed with her glasses on, reading from her Bible. It would make her daughter's day.

Week Twenty-Five

On Thursday morning I went to Room 627 to give Mr. R yet another piece of bad news.

I'd already had to tell him that his foot infection had reached the bone and would require six weeks of IV antibiotics. And that even though he hadn't had a heart attack per se, his heart function was even worse than it had been after his last attack. And, worst of all, I'd told him that his CT scan had picked up a mass in his lung that, along with the enlarged lymph nodes in his chest and abdomen, likely meant that his colon cancer had returned.

Now, to top it off, I was here to report that his gallbladder was enlarged and filled with stones, which were probably causing his stomach pain. Though it was not a surgical emergency, there were signs that sometime in the past the stones had caused bile to back up into his liver and pancreas and would likely do so again soon.

Mr. R was a talker, always warm and effusive but also respectful. Now he looked at me blankly, then said, hesitantly, "Impossible."

At first I thought he'd misunderstood me: I couldn't remember the Spanish for "pancreas" and for the life of me cannot pronounce *hígado* ("liver"). But he looked at his wife for confirmation, and she nodded vigorously. Mr. R told me that he'd had his gallbladder removed in Guatemala more than thirty years ago, then lifted his hospital gown and pointed to a thick, six-inch scar stretching down the right side of his belly.

Though I remembered seeing Mr. R's name at the top of the radiology report, I began to doubt myself. Had I looked at the wrong scan? The only way to be certain was to see for ourselves. I led Mr. R and his wife down the hall on an expedition to the nursing station to get a firsthand look at the computerized images.

By the time we reached the computer, we were all giggling. I pulled up his CT scan and scrolled slowly down to the level of the liver and spleen. And there was the gallbladder, right where it should be, large and lopsided and tucked in tight under Mr. R's liver.

He stared straight at me with twinkling eyes and a barely suppressed smile and declared, "A miracle."

About the author: Jennifer Reckrey MD is a family medicine resident in New York City. Each week while she was an intern, she wrote about her experiences as a brand-new doctor. These stories are from weeks nine and twenty five. "As soon as you have one thing figured out during intern year, you're confronted with something completely different. Sometimes all of these new experiences feel overwhelming. But at other times I'm reminded of why I wanted to be a doctor in the first place."

The women of victoria ward

Muriel Murch
2/6/2009

I remember
The women of Victoria Ward.

The laughter of Liz,
before there were good prostheses
before falsies
left, right or bilateral
were built into the cup size of your choice.
Pacing the corridors
and knitting.
Ready to go home.
Building her strength
with a strand of yarn
Tumbled upwards from the empty cup
against that scarlet scar
beneath the bodice
of her bright summer dress.

I remember
Winnie's eyes
watching feces pour
in a torrent
down her abdomen
searing her flesh
until I bathed her body
changed the bed
and wiped away
her tears.
We named that
foolish pink protuberance
her own John Thomas.
Her slow, shy smile
heralded victory
for the moment.

About the poet: *Muriel (Aggie) Murch RN BSN published* Journey in the Middle of the Road: One Woman's Path through a Mid-Life Education *with Sybil Press in 1995. Her short stories and poetry have appeared in university press and online journals and in three anthologies:* Between the Heart Beats: Poetry and Prose by Nurses *and* Intensive Care: More Poetry and Prose by Nurses, *both published by University of Iowa Press; and* Stories of Illness and Healing: Women Write Their Bodies *(Kent State University Press). Muriel continues to write stories and poetry while concurrently producing a biweekly radio show,* Letter From A. Broad, *for kwmr.org and raising organic blackberries (marinorganic.org) on the farm where she and her husband live.*

About the poem: *"This poem began as an exercise while I was at the Sarah Lawrence Medical Writing work shop a couple of years ago. Poet, teacher and healer John Fox would lead us in our early morning poetry sessions. It did not take long for memories to return and fight for their poetic place on the page."*

wounded messenger

Jèan Howell
2/13/2009

I pulled back the plunger, sucking lidocaine from the bottle into the syringe as I prepared to lance Jimmy's abscess. A voice in my head kept repeating, like a mean-spirited parrot, that I'd never done this procedure before—not even under supervision, and certainly not by myself . . .

I'd met Jimmy two months earlier. He'd come into our clinic with a fever, shortness of breath, a horrible cough, and a crumpled paper photocopy of a chest x-ray taken at another clinic. They'd diagnosed pneumonia and given him a course of antibiotics.

But now a month later, still coughing and drenched in sweat every night, he'd come to see us. He was pale, perspiring, exhausted and in pain. His respiratory rate and pulse were up; his temperature was 100.3.

When I listened to the bottom of his right lung, it sounded as though he were breathing underwater. I excused myself to discuss his case with my supervising physician. We agreed that we needed another chest x-ray as well as some basic labs.

This new film looked just as bad as the previous one. As I stared at it, I noticed thick white shapes where the airways entered the lungs.

"This doesn't look good," Dr. Herman said under his breath. "I'm worried about a mass. See here." He pointed to the white areas. "He needs a CT scan."

This meeting was the beginning of my journey with Jimmy. We treated his pneumonia with more antibiotics, painkillers and cough medicine. We ordered a CT scan; he was scared, but I convinced him to have it done.

As it turned out, he did have a lung mass. Then the biopsy report came back: small-cell carcinoma. Less than two percent of people survive five years after this diagnosis.

I felt an inner protest. Jimmy had quit smoking. He wasn't much older than me. It just wasn't fair.

When I saw Jimmy sitting in an examination room, waiting to hear his CT results, my mind went blank.

"Hi, Jimmy," I squeaked.

"So what's the news? Is it good or bad?" he asked.

I didn't have the guts to tell him, and I wasn't sure it was appropriate for a third-year medical student to do so.

"We'll be with you in a few minutes," I said, feeling like a coward as I went to find Dr Herman.

Jimmy reacted to the news with dead silence. Finally he asked, "So what do we do next?"

He started on chemotherapy. I saw him a number of times over the next few weeks. Once he told me angrily, "This may kill me, but not without a fight. It wasn't invited." He pulled a picture of his five-year-old daughter from his worn leather wallet and told me how much he wanted to be there to watch her grow up.

When he got upset, I'd try to calm him down. I usually ended our visits by saying, "Jimmy, stay strong," thinking that there was no way he could survive . . ..

Now here was his tattooed back, naked in front of me. Again, I felt a sense of protest—he'd lost weight and lost his original teeth, and now he had an abscess under his skin. I tried to focus.

I'd noticed the tattoos in passing before, but now they were staring me in the face. On his right arm was a Maltese Cross with the words "Pecker Wood," and just below his neck was a woodpecker—symbols often associated with white supremacist groups. What kind of person was Jimmy outside of our clinic?

For a few moments, all I could see were these emblems of white supremacy.

I am Cherokee. About five years before meeting Jimmy, I'd spoken to a roomful of people at UC Berkeley about the civil rights and Black Power movements, and not long after that I'd introduced Ralph Nader to a crowd of 800 at UC Davis when he'd campaigned for President on a platform of immigrants' rights and other progressive causes. If Jimmy and I had met under different circumstances, I'd have given him a wide berth.

How would he have reacted to me?

I slipped the needle underneath Jimmy's skin near the abscess, to numb it. Then I plunged the scalpel blade into the abscess center. Usually the skin's resistance gives way and white pus oozes from the incision—but this time, nothing happened.

I dug deeper. Still nothing.

I was relieved that Jimmy couldn't see the sweat beads on my forehead and the dark circles under my armpits.

"I'm just taking some time," I said. "I want to make sure I get it all; I don't want it to give you any more problems."

"That's okay," Jimmy replied.

Then he asked, "Where do you plan on working when you're done with school?"

"I'm not sure yet," I said.

And then he said something unexpected: "I want you to know that I think whatever community you choose to work in will be very lucky to have you. You really care about your patients, and you don't judge them."

There I was, my scalpel buried in his back, uncertain of what I was doing—and Jimmy trusted me. I felt a surge of mixed emotions more intense than any I'd ever known.

I was elated that I'd achieved strong rapport with such a complicated patient; this was the first moment I truly felt like a healer. On the other hand, I wasn't sure I knew what I was doing. And in treating and comforting this particular patient—in fulfilling my duty as a student doctor—wasn't I betraying my other core values?

Just at that moment, the tension under my scalpel gave way, and pus oozed from Jimmy's incision.

About the author: Jèan Howell MD was a medical student in a nine-month rural physician elective when he wrote this. He is currently a family medicine resident at Saint John's Hospital in Saint Paul, Minnesota. Therese Zink MD assisted in the writing of this piece.

see one, do one, teach one

Lisa DeTora
2/20/2009

Back when I was in graduate school and working as a medical writer, a physician told me that the key to learning medical knowledge was simple: see one, do one, teach one. It was a clever (and effective) way of convincing me that I was qualified to teach something—like how to write a report—that I'd only attempted once myself.

Now, on days when nothing goes right, I find myself thinking back to that expression—and to the years when I used to see and do more, before I tried to teach anyone anything.

Soon after college, I worked at a private outpatient facility supervising the care and treatment planning for eighteen developmentally disabled adults. I was, in my own fashion, hoping to make a difference.

My program taught skills that would, we thought, enable our students to enter the workplace. But after years of observing and tracking their progress, I came to understand that most would never hold a job—and that some disabilities outweigh even decades of hard work and incremental improvements.

Some of my class, after taking doses of Haldol or Thorazine on a hot afternoon, would glaze over during group activities. I'd keep an eye on them as they napped in the shade (photosensitivity was a problem) at a table covered with crumbled snacks and third-rate coffee in polystyrene cups.

When overworked higher-ups asked me about this "activity," I'd simply say, "Psychotropic medication makes them sleepy," then go on to dispense markers and faded construction paper to my livelier students.

As my director surveyed us, I could almost hear her mental litany: at least the crayons aren't sitting in puddles of coffee; at least they've taken their meds; at least no one is getting sunburned. At least Lisa's here, making sure that no one's wandering away, getting hurt, spilling coffee or worse.

I had my own "at least" list. At least things are better here than in the old days, I'd tell myself. At least nowadays that nice man with the gold tooth mops the cracked linoleum, even if its dirt is permanently ingrained. At least now the nurses are kind to their charges.

As I roamed the day in a sort of fugue, my job functions shielded me from the pain lurking just out of range. But at night, when I tried to fall asleep, I'd see the scars on women who'd been healthy infants until they were dropped out of windows or thrown against cement walls by unstable adults. Their files hinted at hidden events, stories that would never crystallize. The fragmented notes on their state-mandated records swam before my sleepless eyes.

On the days after these wakeful nights, as if to compensate for the invisible nightmares haunting the files, I would see things that weren't there.

Geraldo Rivera would flash, unbidden and Banquo-like, before my mind's eye as I heated canned spaghetti for my charges, some of whom were survivors of the Willowbrook facility for disabled children, the subject of Geraldo's famous expose.

Nearly twenty years before my time, Geraldo had achieved something—caused something to be done—for some of the people I worked with. What was I doing for them? Could a lunch replete with high-fructose corn syrup atone for the failures of an underfunded mental-health system?

Finally, after seeing just a bit too much, I burned out and fled to graduate school. Looking back, I was trying to move into a more hopeful world, away from the grinding hopelessness of permanent disability.

Gradually, over the course of years, the gritty memories of this job faded, and eventually I got involved in medical matters through research and writing. I no longer did anything directly related to caregiving—no longer fed the disabled or made sure the coffee was fresh—but my modest work reached many more people. I studied and wrote, researched and published.

Today as a college professor, I see my students' faces as they learn to interpret disturbing material—like images of the 1918 influenza pandemic.

My healthy, high-achieving students sometimes find even this distant form of bearing witness unsettling. They're unsure of what to do, to say, to think. Some of them wait for me to tell them what they should be seeing, so that they can get started doing something. I try to teach them to look beneath the surface of their world and seek to understand it a little better before they go on to medical school, law school or other pursuits.

I don't blame them for feeling disturbed by the material, because I find some of it as upsetting as they do. The biggest difference for me now, compared with my younger self, is that I've read a lot about how creating narratives like this one can help to ease trauma by reframing it. I'm not sure how it works, but I like to believe that it does.

My workspace these days is a blend of Victorian architecture, valuable art and piles of well-thumbed books. The coffee cups are biodegradable, and the cookies are fresher than they were back when I "habilitated" people. But I still picture my former charges' gently nodding heads as I do my best to teach my current students well. I perceive that I have followed the arc of seeing, doing and teaching. I saw. I did. And now I teach.

And though my students' thoughts and words sometimes move me to tears, my feelings these days are tempered by the maturity I lacked back when I dished up canned pasta and wiped coffee rings off the tables each afternoon.

About the author: *Lisa DeTora PhD is an assistant professor of English at Lafayette College in Easton, PA, where she teaches Environmental Writing, Medicine and Melodrama in a Global Age and other courses. "I wrote this piece after completing the Advanced Narrative Medicine Workshop at Columbia University's College of Physicians and Surgeons. Because of the work I'd done there, I found myself thinking back to my own experiences in direct care."*

Listening

Elizabeth Szewczyk
2/27/2009

I couldn't erase their words,
catch the breath atoms, stuff
them between lips,
couldn't raise survival rates,
lottery odds dependent on cells suctioned
at the precise moment.

Your chest thumping, frantic,
valves siphoning warmth, drawing
cold through vessels, to your feet
crisping leaves beneath us while
you spoke her life.

Replaying slowly, baby girl, toothless
smile, creative toddler scissoring
Barbie hair (and styling hers to match).
Then, like a runner, sprinting
to that day the tumor revealed
itself, unveiled her future and yours.

You visioned her mane, now extinct,
loose, straight, gracing the crook
of her back, gracing the oval of her
face, strands like gold
embroidery framing emerald eyes.

We'd be mother-friends,
shooting Prom pictures,
scarlet satin shushing past her hips,
his fingers yanking the collar of his tux.
They'd glisten, her upswept hair
perfumed hibiscus.

About the poet: Elizabeth Szewczyk's poems have appeared in Westward Quarterly, Crazylit, Chanterelle's Notebook, Shapes, Sanskrit *and* Freshwater, *which she coedits. She wrote the memoir* My Bags Were Always Packed: A Mother's Journey Through Her Son's Cancer Treatment and Remission *(Infinity Publishing, 2006), detailing her son's successful treatment for Non-Hodgkins Lymphoma. Her first poetry book,* This Becoming, *was published by Big Table Publishing in July 2009. Elizabeth has won the Manchester Community College award in poetry and the Connecticut Celebration of Excellence award for writing. She teaches English at Asnuntuck Community College in Enfield, Connecticut, and lives with her husband Tom and their dogs, Marcus and Sophie.*

About the poem: "This poem was inspired by a friendship that occurred while my fourteen-year-old son Daniel was receiving chemotherapy. I became good friends with another mother whose fifteen-year-old daughter was also being treated for cancer at the same hospital. I wrote the poem when it became evident that this young girl would soon pass away."

miscarriage

Jessica Bloom-Foster
3/6/2009

From the moment I walk into the room, she breaks my heart. She has just been sent to obstetrical triage from the ER, where an ultrasound has revealed a twenty-two-week pregnancy and a cervix dilated to four centimeters—halfway to delivery stage. She is moaning from her labor pains and moving restlessly on the narrow cot.

I am a second-year family medicine resident in a Midwestern hospital, and well past halfway through a busy call night. She is a thin, dusky-skinned woman, and she looks at me with wide, dark eyes full of sadness and pain. Her hair is pulled back with a nylon rag, and most of her front teeth are missing. Her face seems long and gaunt.

I take a rapid history before examining her, noting that she looks far older than her thirty-seven years. She tells me freely that she uses heroin and crack, is in a methadone program and smokes half a pack a day. She has not seen a doctor during this pregnancy. Her pains started at least twenty-four hours ago. This is her eighth child. She has only been using heroin for a few years. I ask her why she started using drugs, but she looks away and shakes her head, unable or unwilling to answer.

The longer we speak, the more difficult I find it to condemn her, despite the damage she has done to herself and her unborn baby; she is so honest and polite, answering me "Yes, ma'am" and "No, ma'am," and her eyes are so full of bottomless guilt. During this brief interview, punctuated by her moans, I keep an eye on the monitors, where I see her contractions coming every few minutes and her baby's heartbeat skittering along at around 150 beats per minute. She says she's feeling a lot of pressure, like she has to go to the bathroom. I put two gloved fingers into her vagina to check her cervix, and I feel no cervix at all but the baby's head, still covered with the slick membrane, pushing back against me.

Then there is a flurry of activity: I call in the nurse and the two other doctors (the fellow and the supervising physician), and the patient is wheeled speedily down to a labor room. Instruments are laid out, lights are turned on. We rush to put on paper gowns and sterile gloves; she is crying and asking if her baby is okay. I try to explain, gently, that the baby is coming too early, that there is nothing we can do to stop her labor now, and that there has never been a baby born this early who has lived.

With a few pushes, this tiny red baby comes out—a boy, the membranes a translucent mask over his face. His eyes are sealed shut, and his heartbeat is visible behind the tiny, bird-like ribcage. Quickly, quickly, I clamp and cut the umbilical cord, pull the membranes from his face and rush him to the nursery to weigh him.

The scale reads 440 grams—less than one pound, confirming that he was born too prematurely to survive. We cover his head with a small, striped knit cap and wrap his cooling body in a blanket like any other baby. It is just a matter of time now— just a matter of waiting for him to die.

I carry him back to the patient's room. She is still lying on the bed with a bright light aimed between her legs, her bottom resting in a pool of amniotic fluid and congealing blood, her legs shaking. The fellow is still waiting for the placenta, so the supervising physician asks if she wants to see her baby.

She nods immediately, tears streaming. But she can only look at him a moment before turning away. When I ask if she wants to hold him, she shakes her head silently.

It is deep in the middle of the night, maybe 3 a.m. The paperwork takes about thirty minutes. I focus on converting the experience of the last half-hour into proper medical terminology and compartmentalizing my emotions until I can get this essential, tedious work done. I've been at work for more than twenty hours, and my neck and shoulders are burning with fatigue and tension. I feel the combination of hunger and nausea that occurs when I stay up most of the night.

Finally I'm caught up. I go to check on the patient. The placenta still isn't out, and the fellow is staying with her while she sits on the toilet, pushing. The fellow tells me to lie down and get some sleep.

I am so grateful for the chance to be alone, use the bathroom, brush my teeth. I lie in the call room, feeling my body's exhaustion and staring at the ceiling, thinking about the woman and her dead baby.

I'm relieved that we didn't try to resuscitate the baby; I know it would have been futile and cruel to try. Yet in my mind I keep seeing the mother's face with its heart-wrenching grief and guilt. And in my hands I keep feeling the insubstantial weight of the baby—and, under my index finger, his heartbeat fading away to cold stillness.

About the author: Jessica Bloom-Foster MD wrote this piece as a journal entry while a family medicine resident. After a stint in private practice in Massachusetts, she was on the clinical faculty of the family medicine residency in Cedar Rapids, Iowa, for several years. In 2009 she moved to Bangor to join the residency faculty at Eastern Maine Medical Center and pursue her interests in integrative medicine and in the medical humanities (not to mention hiking, camping and canoeing). Over the past ten years Jessica has published a smattering of essays and poems: "I have always found writing an essential activity that helps me to record and process the experiences of medical training and practice."

Hard facts and fiction

Brian T. Maurer
3/13/2009

At Daniel's first visit, it had been like pulling teeth to get this fourteen-year-old slip of a boy to talk. Despite my thirty years experience as a physician assistant, I hadn't made much headway. I'd pose a question, and his mother would jump in to answer it. He'd slouched on the exam table, staring at the floor. Occasionally he'd lift his eyes to meet mine, then quickly look away.

Daniel's mother had said she was concerned about him. He didn't sleep at night; he couldn't get up for school. He'd missed so much that he was in danger of failing his grade, and the year wasn't even half over.

Daniel's mother was not much taller than her petite, quiet son. She was dark, slender and attractive, with a blunt, sometimes brusque, manner.

"If you want to know what I think, I think he's depressed—just like his father," she'd said.

I had to agree: Daniel showed many signs of clinical depression.

"We separated last year, and I've filed for divorce," his mother had said. "His dad's a drinker, and he won't get help. It seems like he's powerless to do anything about it."

I couldn't help but wonder what was running through Daniel's mind as he heard these words.

We'd discussed the possibility of trying a prescription medication at the first visit, and Daniel had reluctantly agreed. When I'd seen him again the following week, he'd seemed a bit better.

Today, during our third visit, Daniel almost smiled. He even offered a few words in response to my probing. "He's making progress," I thought as I walked him out to where his mother waited. I asked them to see me in six weeks.

Afterwards, I descended the dimly lit stairwell to our basement lunchroom, feeling emotionally drained. Perhaps my years of clinical practice were beginning to take their toll. Or maybe this quiet boy reminded me of my own struggles with depression during a turbulent adolescence.

After years of putting up with her husband's alcoholism, I mused, Daniel's mother had opted for separation and divorce. I wondered what events and expectations had led to that decision, and how his father's loss might be affecting Daniel's current state. I also wondered what it was like raising Daniel as a single parent.

When I passed the office book-swap box, a title caught my eye: *A Tree Grows in Brooklyn.* I picked it up. Vaguely, I recalled a movie by the same name. I flipped the title page: copyright and first printing, 1943.

That night, temperatures plunged close to zero. Over the weekend I mostly stayed indoors, lying on the parlor sofa with the book. The dog lay at my feet, welcome company while my wife was away for a few days visiting our daughter.

The book turned out to be the story of a second-generation Irish-American family living in Brooklyn at the turn of the twentieth century. The mother works hard to support her husband and two children. The husband gets occasional gigs as a singing waiter through his union, although he can never seem to get ahead—his alcoholism trips him up.

One night the father doesn't come home. On the second day they start looking for him in earnest. A cop discovers him huddled unconscious in a tenement doorway, and he is taken to the hospital. When his wife arrives at the ward, she finds him in a coma, dying from pneumonia. She sits next to his bed, watching over him until he dies.

Later, she argues with the doctor who is filling out the death certificate.

"What are you writing down there—what he died from, I mean."

"Acute alcoholism and pneumonia . . .."

"I don't want you to write down that he died from drinking too much. Write that he died of pneumonia alone."

The parish priest convinces the doctor to acquiesce. The father's age, listed on the death certificate, is thirty-four.

I read steadily into that Sunday evening and took the book to work with me on Monday morning, thinking that I might finish it over lunch.

When I arrived at the office, one of the office staff had laid a chart in the center of the desk blotter with a handwritten note attached. I bent down for a closer look, then slowly dropped into the chair.

It was Daniel's chart. The note said that his father had died of alcoholism over the weekend. He'd passed away in a local hospital ward, his wife at his side.

I flipped through the chart. Daniel's father was thirty-four years old.

Sometimes art mimics life; sometimes it's the other way round.

I left several messages for Daniel on his home answering machine, then sent a card. When I saw him the following week, I learned that he hadn't been back to school since his father's death. Meanwhile, his mother was seeking psychiatric care for herself.

I imagine a page turning and await the next chapter in this struggling family's saga.

About the author: Brian T. Maurer PA-C has practiced pediatric medicine as a physician assistant for the past three decades. As a clinician, he has always gravitated toward the humane aspect of patient care—what he calls the soul of medicine. Over the past decade, Brian has explored the illness narrative as a tool to enhance the education of medical students and to cultivate an appreciation for the delivery of humane medical care. To date he has published two collections of stories, Patients Are a Virtue *and* Village Voices. *He can also be found at his blog, www.briantmaurer.wordpress.com.*

spring

cure

Veneta Masson
3/20/2009

In Latin it means care,
conjures priests and temples
the laying on of hands
sacred pilgrimage
sacrifice
the sickbed
invalid and
solemn attendants.

How far we have come.
Today's English
has neatly expunged
these purely human elements.
Cure is impersonal, consequential
unequivocal, sometimes violent—
the annihilation
of the thing that ails.

This nurse
approaching the patient
has discarded temple garb
for practical scrubs.
His gloved hands
unsheathe the magic bullet,
shoot it through the central line
where it locks onto the target cells.

For the not-yet-cured,
there is still sacred pilgrimage—
that dogged slog
to the high tech shrine,
the health food store,
the finish line of the annual race
where, etched on each undaunted face,
is a gritty tale of survival.

About the poet: *Veneta Masson RN is a nurse and poet living in Washington, DC. She has written three books of essays and poems, drawing on her experiences over twenty years as a family nurse practitioner and director of an inner-city clinic. Information about her poetry collection* Clinician's Guide to the Soul *is available at www.sagefemmepress. com.*

About the poem: "*What started me on the path toward this poem was my ambivalence about symbolic ribbons of all colors, the burgeoning number of annual 'races for the cure' and the question of what the word 'cure' actually means nowadays. Along the way, I was able to clarify my own feelings and deepen my appreciation of the meanings that 'the race' may hold for others.*"

Heart to Heart

Janani Krishnaswami
3/27/2009

I first met you in pre-op. It was my first week as a third-year medical student; my white coat was still white, the hidden interior pockets empty and the ten gel pens neatly tucked in my front pocket still leak-free. Stationed on a surgery rotation, I had officially spent twelve hours in the operating room—a frantic, exhausting blur of standing on tiptoe, gripping surgical retractors and struggling to avoid contaminating the sterile operating field where the surgeons neatly clipped and cut. You were the next case. From your chart I knew the barest facts: your name was Marie; you were forty-five years old, diagnosed with invasive breast cancer and scheduled for surgical removal of both cancer-ridden breasts

As I made my way to meet you, my supervising resident tapped me on the shoulder. "Just to let you know," he said, "you probably won't get much of a history. She only speaks French."

Somewhere among my overworked brain cells lurked a few years' worth of grade-school French, so I shook your hand and launched into what I hoped was a confident introduction. "*Bonjour, Marie! Je suis étudiant en medicine.*" Your eyes lit up, perhaps in recognition of a familiar language, or perhaps in amusement at my rusty *français*—in which I had just referred to myself as a male medical student. Though I could only manage two tenses, we "talked" for the entire hour before your procedure. You were a nurse from Guyana, I learned; a relief organization had covered your travel and medical care. You were nervous—"*un peu*" (a little), you admitted—but also hopeful, ready for what lay ahead.

We spoke but a few complete sentences to each other, yet our conversation left me genuinely invested in your care. I found my sore, sleep-deprived self recharged with enthusiasm as I retracted the muscles in your chest, mentally goaded the surgeons to peel away every cell of cancer, probed your lymph nodes and sutured and cleaned up the surgical wound. As you woke up, I bent down and told you, "*Marie, c'est fini! C'est tout fini!*" (It's finished!)

You were discharged the next day to your host's home. A few weeks later, I took advantage of a day off and phoned up, asking if I might pay a visit. I found you recovering in good spirits; in halting French and English, we talked more about your life in Guyana. I learned further details about the Guyanese refugee program that had constructed the medical and nursing school you had attended—and enabled your care in the U.S. Witnessing this philanthropy in action, I suddenly felt overcome by a sense of déjà vu, the resurfacing of a familiar ideal that had compelled me to become a doctor. It was, quite simply, the promise of making a difference.

You're back in Guyana now, but we've met again this year. Once, you were an Arabic grandmother I encountered in a community free clinic, gripped by fear that you had cancer. You didn't understand my English and I spoke no Arabic. I just held your hand and mouthed "We'll take care of you" over and over; finally you broke into a smile and said in thick, halting English: "I come bring you *muhallabiah*" (a sweet rice pudding). "You will like." Another time, you were the "far gone" patient on the psychiatry ward: a middle-aged woman with a history of substance abuse, bipolar disorder and schizophrenia, who ate only cornflakes and Diet Coke, wandered the locked halls with a guitar and launched into diatribes against doctors, lawyers and men in general. You gazed blankly at me and called me "Sarah," but accepted my gifts of extra cereal boxes (even Cheerios!) with regal grace.

I think of you now as my most important patient. You see, even as the grueling, mundane tasks of residency sometimes strain my idealism, your story renews my commitment to medicine—and that trite but honest goal, making a difference. This goal is reachable, I believe, through adept communication and its healing economies of scale. On an individual level, a doctor's clear and caring message to a patient engenders trust, assuages fears and hastens recovery. Within institutions, physician activism promotes awareness and fosters policy change. In the broader society, education and mentorship through literature, media and government initiatives can bring about real transformation, inspiring the apathetic student or potential drifter to rise as a leader in medicine and beyond.

Marie, I want to thank you. After all, you showed me that the best medium for medicine's healing potential is the language of the heart, and that sometimes the deepest communication and understanding between patient and doctor can come without words.

About the author: Janani Krishnaswami MD graduated from University of Michigan Medical School and is currently a resident in a joint internal medicine/preventive medicine program at Kaiser Permanente and University of California, San Francisco. While at Michigan she regularly contributed to Dose of Reality (www2.med.umich.edu/medschool/reality/), a blog about the medical-school experience, and she is working on publishing a short story on cultural and socioeconomic aspects of medicine in India.

Brain cutting

Emma Samelson-Jones
4/3/2009

The page came to my resident, who grinned and looked over at me, his hovering medical student. "You should go to this."

I looked down at the pager.

"Brain Cutting. 2:30 PM. Room B157."

Text pagers are the indifferent bearers of all news. Emergencies—"Smith, BP 60/30, Room L721"—appear in the same font as messages seemingly borrowed from a teenager's cell phone: "OMG, the harpist in the hospital lobby is playing 'My heart will go on' from Titanic. WTF?"

I dutifully took the elevator down to the hospital basement and opened the door to the morgue. The medical examiner and a group of neurology residents and students were gathered around a steel table, its sides sloping gently down to a central drain.

As more people arrived, the residents repeated the patient's history. Adrenoleukodystrophy—a rare genetic defect, marked by progressive brain damage. Same disease as in that movie *Lorenzo's Oil*. A freak traffic accident involving a train had been followed by worsening weakness. Unsteady gait. Seizures. Personality changes. Death.

Most of the residents had cared for this patient over the previous year. We flipped through a pathology book with autopsy photos of another adrenoleukodystrophy case, then reviewed the brain MRIs that documented our patient's progressive loss of white matter, the myelin sheath insulating the nerves.

"Fascinating," said one student. "Has a case like this one ever been reported in the literature?"

Nobody had seen one; there were plans to write it up.

The medical examiner, a pathologist with long, blond hair pulled back tightly in a low ponytail, reached into a vat of formalin preservative and pulled out a human brain, the spinal cord still attached. She set it on the gleaming table.

Gleeful. The word kept repeating itself in my head as the enthusiasm in the room mounted.

I expected the medical examiner to open a large set of dissection tools to examine the minutiae of this man's brain. Instead, she took out only two instruments: a large, nondescript knife with a ten-inch blade and an industrial-strength metal spatula like those used to flip burgers in restaurants. With clean, confident strokes, she cut half-inch sections, starting at the end of the spinal cord and going all the way up through the brain. After each cut, she scooped up the section with the spatula and lined it up next to the others on the table. Within five minutes, the brain looked like the pictures in the pathology book.

Almost two-and-a-half millennia ago, Hippocrates wrote:

> Men ought to know that from nothing else but the brain come joys, delights, laughter and sports, and sorrows, griefs, despondency, and lamentations. And by this, in an especial manner, we acquire wisdom and knowledge, and see and hear and know what are foul and what are fair, what are bad and what are good, what are sweet, and what are unsavory . . . . And by the same organ we become mad and delirious, and fears and terrors assail us.

Now this essential organ of humanity—the matter underlying the mind, the seat of the soul—was displayed in half-inch sections for us to see.

We took turns feeling how soft the cerebellum's white matter was compared with the rest of the brain.

"Amazing."

"Wow!"

I touched the soft, mushy white matter, thinking about the man, who was apparently funny and kind and unreliable.

The medical examiner, thrilled to have a rapt audience, took the opportunity to teach us how to determine the cause of death for death certificates. Which had killed the patient—the train that had hit him many months earlier, or his disease?

She divided the brain sections into groups: a few sections of the occipital lobe, from the rearmost part of the brain, for a researcher on the East Coast; some spinal-cord sections for a lab in California; the remainder for the local pathology department.

Later, I thought about the relationship between the patient—the man, now dead—and the case, which had lived on in the autopsy specimens and in the glee that had permeated the morgue during the brain cutting.

Is the case a lasting memorial to the deceased? Consider the famous amnesiac HM, whose short-term memory was obliterated by brain surgery. He died last year, but his case lives on in neurology textbooks. Or are the patient and the case two completely separate entities—the case born of the patient as Athena was born of Zeus—once united but ultimately independent, to be examined, discussed and dissected in isolation from one another?

During that hour, as we gleefully dissected the brain of a well-known patient, the case and the patient were separate entities. Perhaps that reflected the ultimate triumph of rationality, of the cortex—the seat of thought and consciousness—over the more emotional limbic system.

Achieving this total disconnect is necessary in some of the work that physicians do. But is a human toll suffered—not by patients such as this man, whose brain was so fascinating that we sent pieces of it to labs across the country, but by the physicians, whose own brain functions become so compartmentalized that they feel no empathic response?

About the author: *Emma Samelson-Jones MD is a psychiatry resident at Columbia University. "I went to medical school because I wanted to 'be of use' and because I was interested in people's stories. Physicians have incredible access to the lives of individuals, which is what keeps me excited about coming back to the hospital. Nonfiction writing is a way for me to sort out my own ideas and to share them with a wider audience."*

mistaken identity

Kathleen Grieger
4/10/2009

Surgery finished,
I finally sleep

Pushing my shoulders,
the technician wakes me

"Come now, we need
a chest x-ray"

Smiling, she pulls me
into position

The x-ray machine
tight against me

Finally getting a chance,
I ask what she is doing

"Oh," she says "I have
the wrong one

You are not a 64
year old male"

Lying me down,
she walks away

As I fall back to sleep,
I wonder, now bald

what I must
look like

About the poet: *Kathleen Grieger has published poetry in many venues, including* Free Verse, Caduceus, Blood and Thunder: Musings on the Art of Medicine, The Healing Muse *and online in* Yale Journal for Humanities in Medicine *and* Breath and Shadow. *She has written hundreds of poems about her brain surgeries as well as her interactions with physicians and other healthcare professionals. Her poems are currently used at Froedtert Hospital in Milwaukee to teach that patients are people first.*

About the poem: "*Frustrated with the problems and errors that were hugely complicating my medical treatment after brain surgery, I realized that it was necessary for me to start writing again. Because I'd been so busy before, my poetry had been set aside; picking it up again was the best thing I've ever done.*"

coming full circle

Stacy Nigliazzo
4/17/2009

Only thirty minutes into my evening ER nursing shift, and I was already behind. My first patient was a pregnant teenager with heavy vaginal bleeding. "About three months, I guess," she flatly replied when asked about her last period. As we placed her legs in the stirrups for the pelvic exam, torrents of blood and water rolled into the kick bucket on the floor.

Dr. Parkman had barely opened the speculum when we saw it. I knew she couldn't see the doctor's face, but she could see mine. Shielding her from my expression, stunned and speechless, I cowered as best I could behind her left knee.

There it was. Tiny, pink and perfect. Her baby's hand, so small that it would easily fit inside the shell of a walnut—outstretched as if reaching for us, for its very life.

The doctor and I both instantly knew there was no chance of survival. It just wasn't time yet. He removed the speculum, and we watched as the tiny fingers slowly disappeared back inside.

Fifteen minutes later I exited the labor and delivery floor with an empty stretcher, having left my patient in a stark delivery room, pushing. The screeching fetal heart monitor echoed throughout the unit. I paged the chaplain and the social worker to come help her face the grim reality of her child's certain death. I wanted to give her more, but in my heart I knew that we could provide only comfort and support. It would be cruel to offer any hope that this infant would live.

I returned to the ER and found her former room already prepared for the next patient, en route to us via ambulance. My charge nurse gave me the report: ninety-seven-year-old female from a nursing home, generalized weakness. I would have taken the Lord's name in vain then and there, but I didn't have time. I knew all too well the grueling amount of care she'd likely need—and I'd also been assigned three other patients while I was gone.

I hardly had time to make rounds on them and to gather the necessary equipment before she arrived, her presence announced by the clanking squeal of a rolling metal stretcher. I could barely make out her tiny form beneath a big pile of gray blankets.

"No family to speak of; she's pretty much outlived them all," said the paramedic, handing me her medical chart. I opened it and was puzzled to see no daily medications or previous diagnoses listed. I wondered if it was really possible for someone to walk this earth for close to a century without a scratch. One could only hope.

Somewhat skeptically, I introduced myself and awaited her reply. Her gentle eyes instantly captivated me; I was eager to hear her voice.

She told me her name was "Mrs. Jack Winston" and confirmed what her chart indicated. Her warm, welcoming manner and quiet eloquence charmed me. "I don't see my doctor too often, but she's a dandy, all the same," she remarked.

I asked her about shortness of breath, chest pain and every other ominous symptom I could think of. One by one, she denied them all. I stood still beside her, confused and fascinated.

After a few quiet moments of thought, I gathered up the monitoring equipment and started to record her vital signs. Carefully, I peeled away the blanketed layers to reveal her frail, emaciated frame.

She was wearing a simple white nightgown that sheathed her arms down to the fingertips. She looked like an angel. Ethereal, almost. Preparing to take her blood pressure, I folded back her left sleeve.

There it was. Withered, wrinkled and weather-beaten. Her hand, adorned with the same silver band she'd worn every day for the last sixty years, even though the man who first placed it there had died nearly twenty years ago.

Trembling, she reached for me as if for her very life. I leaned in closer and, taking her hand in both of my own, tightly embraced it.

She smiled and whispered, "Honey, this old body's been very good to me, but I'm tired. It's just time."

About the author: Stacy Nigliazzo RN is an ER nurse and a lifelong poet. Her work has been featured in Pulse, Creative Nursing, American Journal of Nursing, Blood and Thunder and Penn State International Journal of Healthcare and Humanities. She is a graduate of Texas A&M University and is a 2006 recipient of the Elsevier award for nursing excellence.

indexes

index by author

Poems

index by title, with summaries

Stories

index by healthcare role

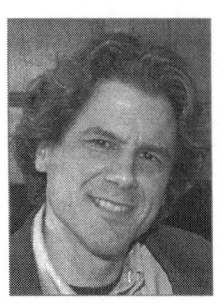

Paul Gross is founding editor of the online magazine *Pulse—voices from the heart of medicine*. He is an assistant professor in the Department of Family and Social Medicine at Albert Einstein College of Medicine and Montefiore Medical Center in the Bronx, where he teaches narrative medicine. His stories about medical practice and family life have appeared in *American Family Physician, Journal of Family Practice, Hippocrates, The Sun, Diversions* and *Town & Country*. He has also conducted award-winning writing workshops for medical professionals.

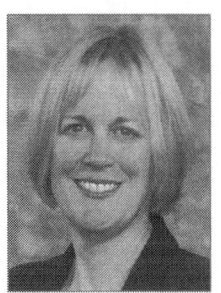

Diane Guernsey is executive editor of *Pulse—voices from the heart of medicine*. Formerly a senior editor at *Town & Country Magazine*, she is still a *T&C* contributor, writing about health, medicine and other topics. Her professional interests embrace several fields: she performs as a classical pianist and is on the faculty of Manhattanville College in Purchase, NY, as a piano instructor, vocal coach and accompanist; and she is also a licensed psychoanalyst with a small practice in Manhattan.

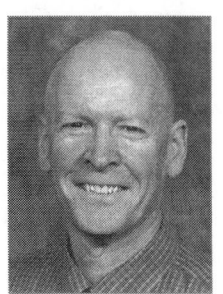

Peter Selwyn is chairman of the Department of Family and Social Medicine, and professor of Family Medicine and Internal Medicine, at Montefiore Medical Center and Albert Einstein College of Medicine in the Bronx, New York. He is also the founder and director of the Palliative Care Service at Montefiore Medical Center. Dr. Selwyn authored *Surviving the Fall: the Personal Journey of an AIDS Doctor* (Yale University Press,1998), which was nominated for the National Book Award. He has researched and published widely on HIV/AIDS, substance abuse, underserved populations and palliative care.

Made in the USA
Charleston, SC
16 January 2012